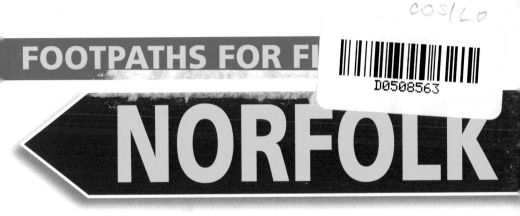

FOOTPATHS FOR F[I]

NORFOLK

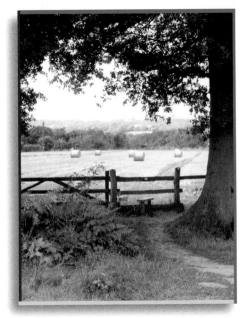

Anita Delf and
Marilyn Taylor

COUNTRYSIDE BOOKS

NEWBURY BERKSHIRE

First published 2008
© Anita Delf and Marilyn Taylor, 2008

COUNTRYSIDE BOOKS
3 Catherine Road
Newbury, Berkshire

To view our complete range of books,
please visit us at
www.countrysidebooks.co.uk

ISBN: 978 1 84674 091 6

Cover picture supplied by
David Weller

Maps by CJWT Solutions
Photographs by Marilyn Taylor

Designed by Peter Davies, Nautilus Design
Produced through MRM Associates Ltd., Reading
Printed by Information Press, Oxford

CONTENTS

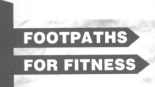

FOOTPATHS FOR FITNESS

FOOTPATHS FOR FITNESS

GRADE 1 – STROLL

WALK ❶ CASTLE ACRE... 8
Off We Go! *¾ mile*

WALK ❷ BLICKLING.. 12
Walking With A Queen *1¼ miles*

WALK ❸ SANDRINGHAM ESTATE 17
A Royal Outing *1 mile*

WALK ❹ WYMONDHAM 21
An Abbey To Behold *1½ miles*

WALK ❺ BURSTON 26
Pupil Power *2 miles*

WALK ❻ WHITLINGHAM COUNTRY PARK 30
A Mustard Legacy *2½ miles*

FOOTPATHS FOR FITNESS

GRADE 2 – STRIDE

WALK ❼ HORNING 34
Ahoy There! *3 miles*

WALK ❽ OXBOROUGH 38
A National Treasure *3¼ miles*

WALK ❾ REEDHAM 42
Views Galore! *3½ miles*

WALK ❿ MATTISHALL 46
'Nosy Parker' Was Here *3½ miles*

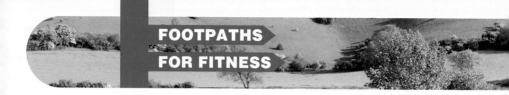

FOOTPATHS FOR FITNESS

WALK ⑪ SHOTESHAM 50
A Picture-Postcard Stride *4 miles*

WALK ⑫ FAKENHAM 54
A Printer's Paradise *4 miles*

WALK ⑬ REEPHAM 58
A Churchyard For Three *4½ miles*

WALK ⑭ HICKLING BROAD 62
Nature Lovers' Delight *4 miles*

WALK ⑮ THE BURNHAMS 67
Naval Salute *4 miles*

WALK ⑯ WINTERTON-ON-SEA 72
Giants Abound *5 miles*

WALK ⑰ TERRINGTON ST JOHN 77
Wide Skies and Open Spaces *5 miles*

FOOTPATHS FOR FITNESS

GRADE 3 – HIKE

WALK ⑱ BLAKENEY 81
Rarin' To Go! *7 miles*

WALK ⑲ WEETING CASTLE AND GRIME'S GRAVES 85
Shifting Up a Gear! *7½ miles*

WALK ⑳ HOUGHTON, HARPLEY AND PEDDARS WAY 90
Fit As A Fiddle! *8½ miles*

Introduction

Walking is recognised as an excellent way of promoting physical fitness. It is also a pleasurable and low cost activity. We both came to walking relatively late in life. With more time for ourselves as our families demanded less of us, we wanted to do something that would increase our fitness levels, help us lose weight and be of low cost but also pleasurable. Walking met all these requirements and now, 15 years later, we are continuing to enjoy all the benefits that walking brings.

In this book, which has been a pleasure to write, we have started with short gentle walks, gradually increasing their length and the degree of challenge so that in time you will be encouraged to progress to the longer walks. Each walk is circular, apart from Walk 7, with points of interest added along the way to keep up your enthusiasm.

Walking has made us stronger and healthier, it has also increased our mental well being. The joy of walking is difficult to describe, everyday stresses seem to melt away with each stride. For us the delights of spotting different birds and wild flowers, and exploring ancient churches and landmarks never diminishes. The Norfolk landscape is incredibly varied, you can walk through an open landscape with its huge expanse of blue skies, explore the Broads National Park, go amongst the forests of Breckland or enjoy any of the villages and market towns.

We have walked our favourite walks many times, whilst new walks bring new discoveries and delights. The timings given should be seen as a guide as people have differing stride lengths and walk at different speeds.

We have tried to ensure that most of the walks are accessible by public transport, however, as these walks are mainly in rural areas the transport is often limited or seasonal. The following telephone numbers should be able to supply details of the services available: 'One' railway 0845 600 7245 and First Eastern Bus Company 01603 788306.

A camera and binoculars, if you have them, can add to the pleasure of the walk. Walking boots are recommended as they give necessary ankle support, especially on rough ground and they are waterproof. They can be found in any reputable outdoor equipment specialist who will be pleased to give help and advice, and once purchased will last for some years. Trainers or comfortable shoes can be used on the shorter walks if the ground is dry underfoot. Wear loose clothing and if the weather forecast is not good take a hat and a lightweight coat, the lighter the better. Breathable lightweight jackets are excellent. A backpack is useful for carrying extra clothing and a bottle of water with you on the walks. For those of a longer length we recommend you also take a snack. A pedometer can be useful for calculating the distance walked.

Happy walking!

Anita Delf and Marilyn Taylor

Publisher's Note

We hope that you obtain considerable enjoyment from this book; great care has been taken in its preparation. Although at the time of publication all routes followed public rights of way or permitted paths, diversion orders can be made and permissions withdrawn.

We cannot, of course, be held responsible for such diversion orders and any inaccuracies in the text which result from these or any other changes to the routes, nor any damage which might result from walkers trespassing on private property. We are anxious though that all details covering the walks are kept up to date and would therefore welcome information from readers which would be relevant to future editions.

The simple sketch maps that accompany the walks in this book are based on notes made by the author whilst checking out the routes on the ground. They are designed to show you how to reach the start, to point out the main features of the overall circuit and they contain a progression of numbers that relate to the paragraphs of the text.

However, for the benefit of a proper map, we do recommend that you purchase the relevant Ordnance Survey sheet covering your walk. The Ordnance Survey maps are widely available, especially through booksellers and local newsagents.

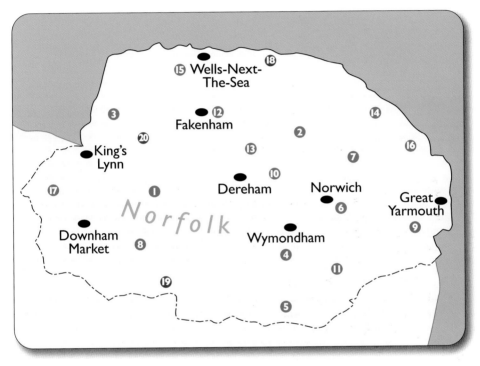

Area map showing location of the walks

Grade 1 – STROLL

Grade 2 – STRIDE

Grade 3 – HIKE

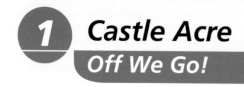

1 Castle Acre

Off We Go!

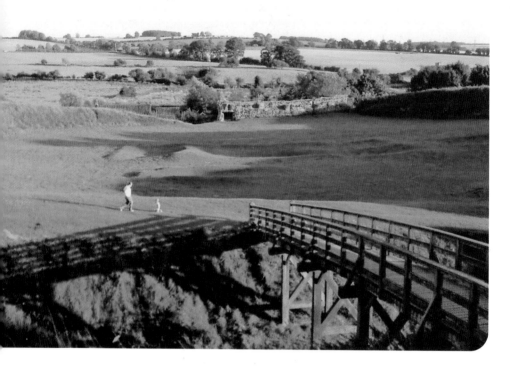

■ *Looking down from the castle ruins* ■

If you are new to walking, and we all have to start somewhere, then this is a wonderful place to begin. Castle Acre, surrounded by lovely countryside, has fine buildings and a wealth of historic interest. On this walk, which circles the village centre, you can visit the ruins of the castle and take a peep at the remains of the Cluniac Priory, both of which are maintained by English Heritage. There are information boards which tell of the castle's history.

GRADE: 1
ESTIMATED CALORIE BURN: 75

Terrain: Mainly flat, short section uphill to the castle.
Distance: ¾ mile
Stiles: None
Time: 45 minutes, including exploring the castle ruins
Starting point: Stocks Green. GR 816152 (roadside parking)
How to get there: Castle Acre is 4 miles north of Swaffham, off the A1065 Swaffham to Fakenham road.
OS map: Explorer 236 King's Lynn, Downham Market and Swaffham
Refreshments: The village boasts two good public houses with eateries, a local shop selling good picnic fare and the Willow tea room – one of the best teashops in Norfolk.

The castle was constructed by Earl William de Warenne, son-in-law of William the Conqueror, now only the 11th-century bailey gateway and earthworks remain. The castle has wonderful views overlooking the River Nar, which clearly show the strength of its position. The village green was once part of the outer castle bailey but is now surrounded by a charming mix of houses and shops. This is where the stocks would have been situated, in a time when public punishment was the norm. So take a walk around this pretty village, originally a small medieval walled town, and enjoy all it has to offer, including a visit to the priory which was built for the Cluniac order of France and is attributed to the son of William de Warenne. The abbey was originally sited within the castle precincts, but was soon moved to its present position. Its ruins span 7 centuries and include a 15th-century gatehouse, a 12th-century church with a much-photographed west front and a prior's lodging. The priory once housed the severed arm of St Phillip and in medieval times a constant flow of pilgrims came to the see the relic hoping for cures. Their gifts helped to make the priory wealthy. The last prior signed it away to Henry VIII in 1537.

Walkers are a common sight in Castle Acre, as The Nar Valley Way, running from King's Lynn to Dereham, goes through the village and it is also the crossing point for the Peddars Way National Trail.

1 Walk along **Stocks Green** with the Ostrich public house on the right. Continue towards the parish church passing the Willow tea room on the left, continue beyond it and go through the gateway of the churchyard. The

9

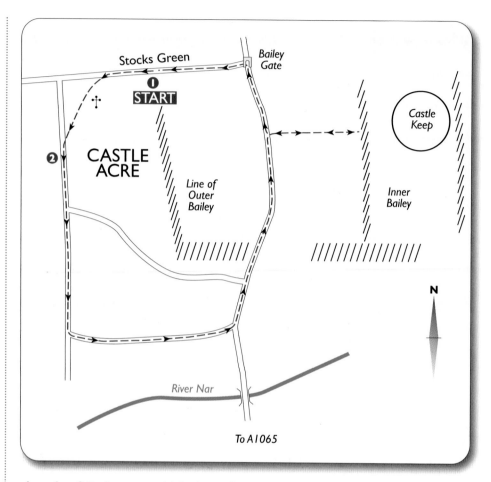

church of St James, which dates from the 13th century, stands upon the site of an earlier building and its interior is worthy of a visit. Walk diagonally right to the churchyard exit in the far corner, go down the steps and turn left along the lane.

2 Continue along the lane, passing Chimney Street on the left, then take the next left along **Blind Lane**. At its end keep left and turn left onto a country road, passing **Cuckstool Lane** on the right. This is a reminder of past punishments when a cuck or ducking stool would have operated here. Loose, vulgar, drunken women or scolds would have been strapped into a chair and plunged into the river to shame them into behaving. Continue to walk uphill along **Bailey Street** with its picturesque houses, then just before

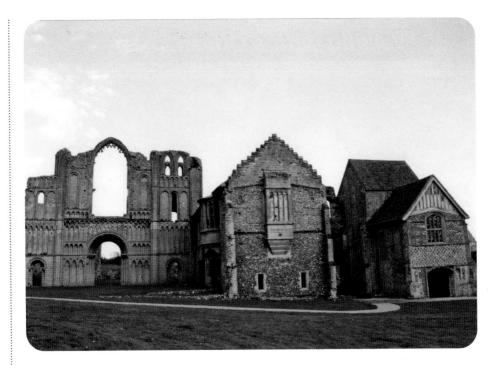

■ *Castle Acre priory* ■

the **Old Red Lion House**, turn right to follow a gravel track into the grounds of the castle. After exploring the site, retrace your steps to the road and turn right towards the 13th-century Bailey Gate, going through the gate which has portcullis grooves between its arches, then turn left back onto **Stocks Green** and the end of the walk.

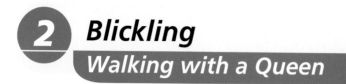

2 Blickling

Walking with a Queen

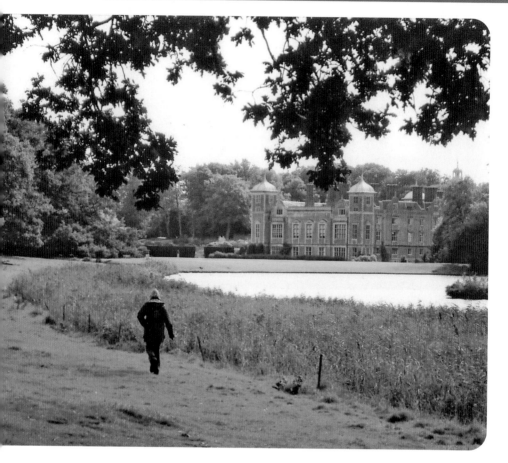

■ *In the grounds of Blicking Hall* ■

This delightful walk in the grounds of the National Trust's Blickling Hall, is lovely in any season. There are no stiles and the walk is an easy route around the lake and through the extensive parkland on good marked paths, with the added bonus of Blickling Hall and its fascinating history.

The hall is a truly magnificent building, its visual impact is outstanding, whether seeing it for the first or fiftieth time. It is said to be one of the finest examples of Jacobean architecture in the country. It was left to the National Trust in 1940 after the death of Lord Lothian, whose family had owned it since 1850. It was opened to the public in 1962 following restoration. The Jacobean hall is the work of architect Robert Lyminge, who also designed Hatfield House. His employer, Sir Henry Hobart, purchased the then dilapidated hall in 1616. The first house on the site had belonged to King Harold, then a moated hall was built in the 14th century. By 1505 it had passed into the hands of the Boleyn family and it is believed Anne Boleyn was born there. It is said that the headless ghost of Queen Anne still haunts the property. Robert Lyminge incorporated some of the medieval house into his new design for the wonderful Jacobean hall we see today.

In the concert area highly popular musical events take place over a series of summer evenings. There have been many artists performing in recent years. An evening of popular classical music *The Last Night of the Proms* – is a particular favourite of many. Concert-goers bring elaborate picnics with tables, chairs, even a candelabra, as they enjoy this magical experience.

Behind the centre is Samphire, an award-winning shop selling organic local produce and gifts. Celebrity chef, Gary Rhodes, declared the speciality rare-breed sausages to be 'the best' he had ever tasted. Royal Air Force personnel were billeted at Blickling Hall during the course of the Second World War and there is a fine display relating to the role of RAF Oulton in the room adjacent to the tea room. There are plant sales in the courtyard and beyond those is the Lothian Barn. This beautifully restored barn houses a most amazing collection of second-hand books, covering a vast range of subjects, enter only if you have lots of time at your disposal!

GRADE: 1
ESTIMATED CALORIE BURN: 110

Terrain: Flat, well maintained footpaths.
Distance: 1¼ miles
Stiles: None
Time: 1 hour
Starting point: National Trust visitors' car park (fee payable). GR 175286.
How to get there: Blickling Hall is off the B1354, 1 mile north-west of the market town of Aylsham. It is well signposted.
OS Map: Landranger 133
Refreshments: Excellent National Trust tea room at the hall or the Buckinghamshire Arms public house in Blickling village.

1 From the car park walk, in the direction of the visitor centre. Follow the signpost by the visitor centre to the park and lake and go through the wooden fence, turn right and continue along the tarmac lane in the direction of the **Buckinghamshire Arms**. Before reaching it, however, turn

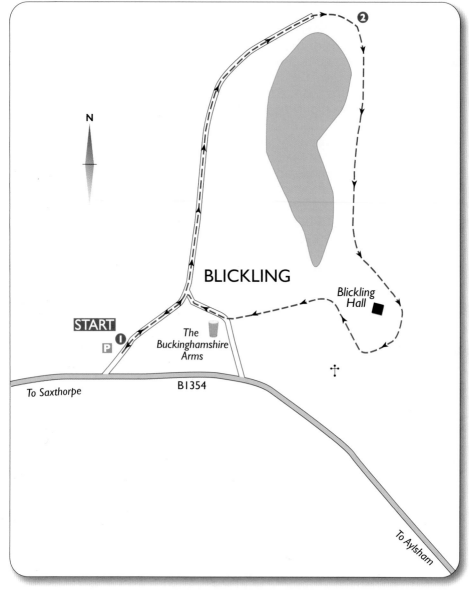

N

2

BLICKLING

Blickling Hall

START

P **1**

The Buckinghamshire Arms

B1354

To Saxthorpe

To Aylsham

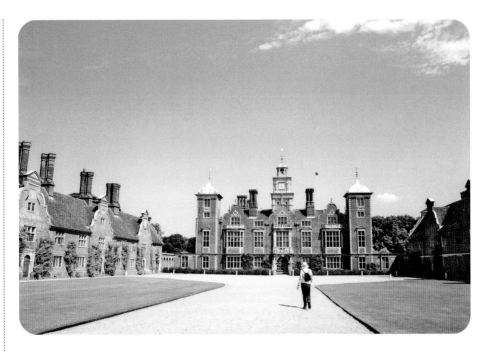

■ *The magnificent frontage of the hall* ■

left at the sign for the **Lakeside Walk**. Turn left again after a few yards at the sign 'to lake and park'. Go through a wooden gate with the sign 'dogs on leads'. Dogs are welcome on the Blickling estate, however, there may be cattle grazing so a lead is advisable. Continue ahead through the trees and soon the west wing of Blickling Hall will become visible, this gives a stunning view as you follow the path towards the lake.

2 Go through the wooden gate continuing with the lake on the right, you are now in the concert area. Pass through another gate still following the path around the lake. As you follow the path away from the lake there is a wonderful view of the rear of the hall which, viewed from any angle, never looks less than breathtaking. Continue on the footpath going through a further gate, stock may be grazing here, but the cattle are so accustomed to walkers that they take no notice of anyone. Maintain direction passing through the next gate, parts of the superb gardens can be seen to the right enticing a visit. Go through a further gate and continue ahead. On the right is a temple built in 1773 and now sometimes used for wedding ceremonies. The walk passes by an orangery built by Samuel Wyatt in 1782; wedding ceremonies are also held in this wonderful setting. The next and last gate leads past the **Old Vicarage** on the left. Walk either from the courtyard, or the tea room to the gravel drive fronting the hall, flanked on either side by an outstanding yew hedge. The truly superb frontage is visible for the first time on the walk. The hedges are cut from August to mid October. The yew cuttings are collected to make a cancer-fighting drug. Turn right at the end of the drive and follow the path round to the right passing the **Buckinghamshire Arms**. Known locally as 'the Bucks', it was built in 1693 as a coaching inn and housed both guests and servants from the hall. From the Buckinghamshire Arms turn left back to the car park.

3 Sandringham Estate
A Royal Outing

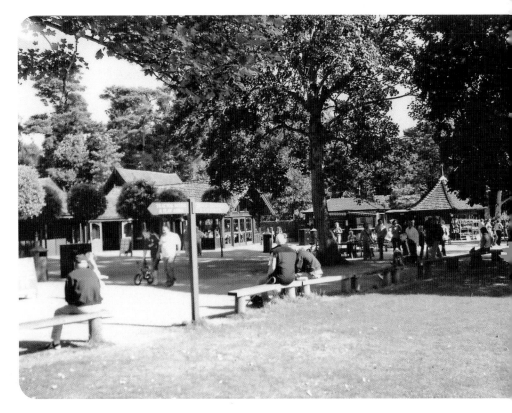

■ *The shops and refreshment area at Sandringham* ■

he country park of the royal estate of Sandringham is ideal for walking. Set within the Norfolk Coast Area of Outstanding Natural Beauty, it is open daily and provides excellent walking at any time of the year. Although visited by many, the woodland park maintains a very quiet atmosphere with plenty of wildlife to enjoy. There are marked trails through the woodland and we have chosen to follow the blue trail for this short walk, which begins and ends at the Visitor Centre. There is a small play area for children. Dogs on leads are allowed in the park.

Sandringham has been a royal estate since its purchase by Queen Victoria in 1862 for her eldest son, the Prince of Wales, later to be King Edward VII.

17

GRADE: 1
ESTIMATED CALORIE BURN: 100

Terrain: Flat sandy tracks with tarmac estate roads.
Distance: 1 mile
Stiles: None
Time: 45 minutes
Starting point: The visitor centre, Sandringham Estate Country Park. GR 690288.
How to get there: Sandringham Country Park is off the A149 coast road just south of Dershingham. Follow the brown tourist signs and then the car parking signs on entering. Parking is free.
OS Map: Explorer 250 Norfolk Coast West
Refreshments: The visitor centre has a range of refreshments. There is also plenty of space for picnics.

The original house, considered too small, was replaced by the Jacobean style building familiar to us from coverage of the Queen's annual Christmas message. Sandringham House has been open to the public since 1977 and the Country Park covers over 600 acres. The entire estate stretches for more than 7,000 acres and encompasses seven parishes, there is, however, no village of Sandringham.

There is no charge to visit the church, which is highly ornate with a solid silver altar and reredos. It is often seen on television at Christmas time when the Royal family attend services whilst in residence at Sandringham House. Tractor tours will take you round the estate, and an entrance fee is charged to visit the house and beautiful gardens. This is subject to restriction if Sandringham House is in use, although the park is always open for visitors.

1 Walk to the visitor centre, sign posted from the car park. From there follow the signs to the play area, then take the path with the play area and the large grasshopper sculpture on the right. Continue between the tall sculptures of a bear and a raven. The trails are marked with blue or yellow paint on trees. Continue ahead, you will see a trail board on the right at ground level, the blue trail is 1 mile, the yellow trail is 2 miles. This walk follows the **blue trail**.

Keep ahead as directed by the blue arrows on the trees, the trail goes through rhododendron bushes before emerging on to a large grassy avenue, turn right as indicated by two blue arrows on the tree to the right. Turn and

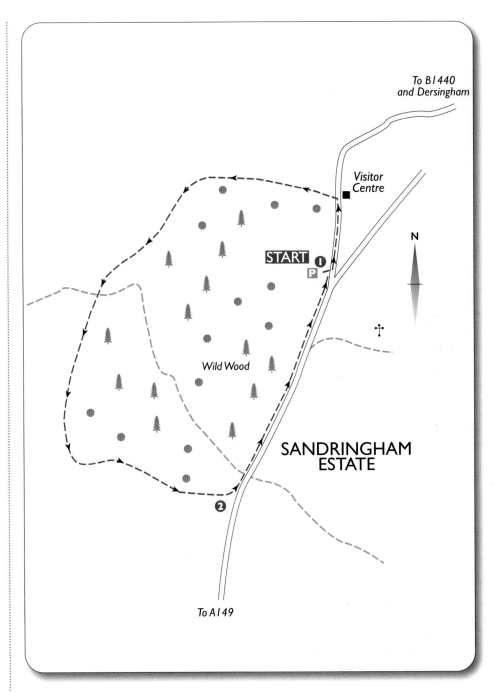

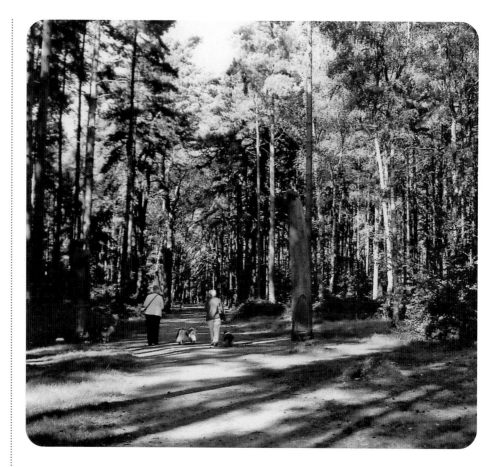

■ *On the route* ■

look back at the view of the wide grassy avenue as it stretches back to the area of the visitor centre. Walk ahead to arrive at the long straight estate road, turn left along it and walk until you reach a tall wooden post with a trail board with blue and yellow arrows painted on it.

2 Turn left, as instructed, then maintain direction at the trail crossroads, passing a wooden sculpture of a mermaid. A further 75 yards beyond the sculpture, turn left along the trail at the blue arrow sign. Shortly after this the trail leads towards an estate road which can be seen through the trees. Turn left again, however, as directed, before reaching the road. Continue to follow the trail to arrive back at the large grassed area near the visitor centre.

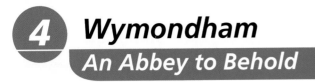

4 **Wymondham**
An Abbey to Behold

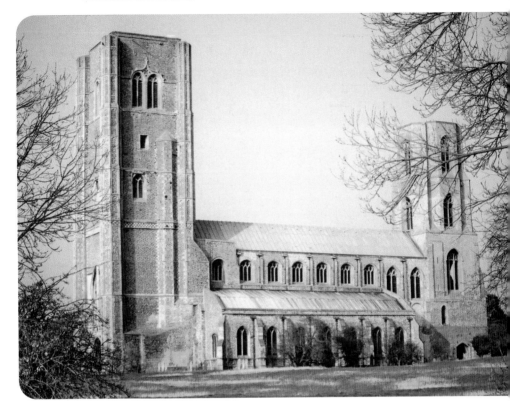

■ *Wymondham Abbey* ■

Wymondham **with its medieval streets**, market cross and great abbey is a delightful town, full of interest for this short walk. The route takes you to the abbey, whose two towers dominate the countryside for miles around, and follows a stretch of the River Tiffey. The river is at the heart of a countryside project to restore meadowland, thereby encouraging a diverse mixture of wildlife.

The church, when built, was intended for use by both the Benedictine monks and the parishioners of Wymondham; however, arguments ensued over who had rights to which part and the priory took over. The parishioners refused to cede to the priory and even the intervention of the Pope failed

> **GRADE: 1**
> **ESTIMATED CALORIE BURN: 150**

Terrain: Flat walking along town streets and riverside paths.
Distance: 1½ miles
Stiles: None
Time: 1 hour
Starting point: Pay and display car park, Market Street. GR 109016. Follow town centre signs, the car park is on the left just beyond the Market Cross
How to get there: Wymondham is off the A11 nine miles south-west of Norwich.
OS Map: Landranger 144
Refreshments: Several possibilities, including the Green Dragon public house which is close to the beginning of the walk. For something different, try Brief Encounter, an award-winning coffee shop and restaurant at Wymondham railway station.

to bring lasting agreement. The replacement of the Norman tower by the monks in 1376 and their annexing of the town bells for their own tower fuelled the quarrel and it was left to Henry VI to arrange a compromise again. The townspeople were still unhappy and sought permission for a new tower for their own bells. This was finally built in the 15th century. The dissolution of the monasteries led to the destruction of much of the priory buildings, but its tower remains for us to enjoy today. There are excellent guides to its history inside the abbey and it is well worth a visit.

Weaving and woodturning were once the main industries of Wymondham. Damgate Street has fine examples of the weavers' cottages. Horsehair weaving continued into the 20th century, whilst the production of small wooden objects continued until the 1980s. The nearby village of Spooner Row owes its name to the spoon-making industry of the Middle Ages. Wymondham also had major brush-making factories.

The walk goes to the Victorian cemetery before returning via Damgate Street and its ancient houses to its start. On your return, do visit the Wymondham Heritage Museum in the old Bridewell to find out more about Robert Kett, a son of Wymondham and leader of the 1549 Kett Rebellion, and the continuing existence of Kett's Oak. Robert Kett owned land close to Becketswell. Following his defeat he was hanged from Norwich Castle and his brother William was hanged from the great west tower of the abbey.

1 From the car park enter **Market Street** and turn left. If you look along the street to the right you will see the Market Cross, constructed in 1616. It now houses the Tourist Information Centre. Continue to Church Street and turn left again. This passes the Chapel of Thomas à Becket, founded by William D'Albini after the Norman Conquest. He also founded the priory which was later to become Wymondham Abbey. Most of the present chapel dates from 1400. Continue, passing the **Green Dragon** pub which dates from the late 15th century. Fortunately this superb building survived the great fire of 1615, when 327 families lost their property. The fire started in a stable whilst many people were in church. Follow the road, with its many attractive houses, then enter the abbey churchyard. Leave the churchyard through the gate by the north porch and turn left onto **Becketswell Road**, continue ahead over the bridge and turn left through the kissing gate to the Riverside Walk at the Becketswell sign. On the right along Becketswell Road is the car park and entrance to the Abbey Halt station of the Mid Norfolk Railway. This organisation, established in 1995, has restored the line

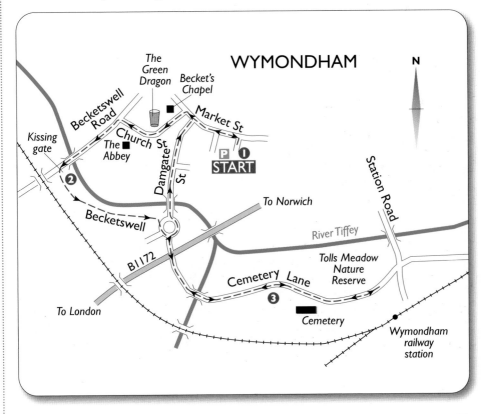

23

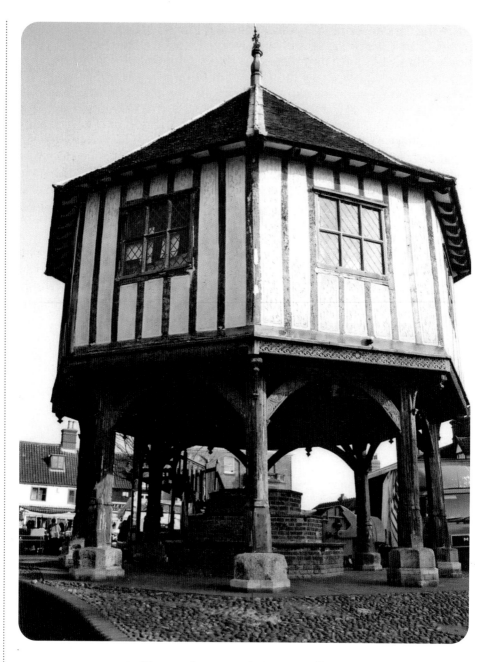

■ *The market cross in Wymondham* ■

running between East Dereham and Wymondham and has plans for further restoration. It carries goods and equipment destined for the armed forces at Swanton Morley.

2 Continue ahead along Becketswell, with the **River Tiffey** on the left, to reach Damgate Street. There are amazing views of the abbey as you walk along Becketswell, which was restored by the Wymondham Town Council in the early 1990s as a much-appreciated recreational area. Turn right at Damgate Street, which becomes Whitehorse Street as you walk along, and continue to the main road. Cross this with care to **Cemetery Lane** opposite and continue down this lane to visit the Victorian cemetery. If you are ready to walk a little further you could continue to the Brief Encounter restaurant and tea room. Follow the signs to Wymondham railway station.

3 From the cemetery (or restaurant) retrace your steps to **Damgate Street** and walk along this to Market Street at the end, then turn right to return to the start.

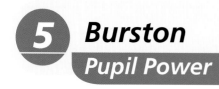

5 Burston

Pupil Power

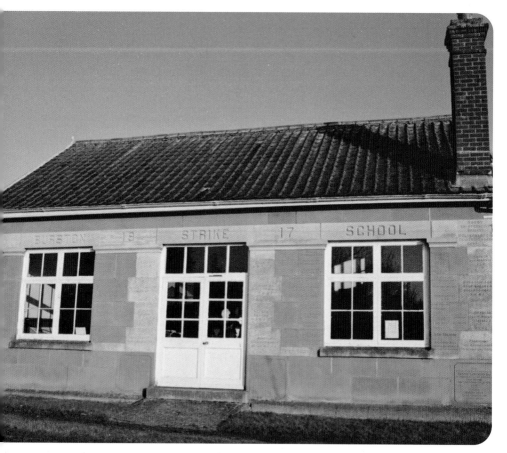

■ *Burston Strike School Museum* ■

This is an easy route, just a little longer than the first walks, around the pretty village of Burston in south Norfolk. In this unlikely setting began the longest strike in history and brought this village fame. Its story is told in the Burston Strike School Museum situated on Church Green where this walk begins and ends.

Tom and Kitty Higdon were the headmistress and senior teacher of the local school but their views on education led them into direct conflict with

GRADE: 1
ESTIMATED CALORIE BURN: 160

Terrain: Flat country lanes and footpaths.
Distance: 2 miles
Stiles: 2
Time: 1½ hours
Starting point: The Burston Strike School Museum car park on Church Green, where there is free car parking. GR 137831.
How to get there: Burston is on a minor road 2 miles west of the A140, 18 miles south of Norwich and 3 miles north-east of Diss.
OS Map: Explorer 230 Diss and Harleston
Refreshments: The Crown public house, Crown Green.

its local management committee. Matters came to a head in 1914 when the managers engineered their dismissal by dubious means. The pupils, however, had other ideas. Led by 13-year-old Violet Potter and supported by their parents they went on strike! It is a measure of the inspiration the Higdons engendered that the parents of the pupils remained firm against the landowners and employers alike, who ransacked their property, destroyed their allotments and threatened them with eviction. Of the school's 72 pupils, 66 were involved in the strike. Lessons were initially taken outside, then a carpenter's shop was rented, until finally a new purpose-built school was erected and opened by Violet Potter in 1917. Donations for the building of this school were sent from all over the United Kingdom. The strike school was finally closed following the death of Tom Higdon in 1939, 25 years after the strike began. The Strike School Museum can be visited during daylight hours. Instructions for the key are posted on the door.

1 Walk to the road from the museum and turn left, passing St Mary's church on the left. Tom and Kitty Higdon are buried here. Turn left into **Mill Road** and then turn right going along the drive of the **Crown public house**. Turn left down a narrow alleyway at the yellow waymark sign of the Norfolk County Council, going between buildings, and passing the Old Pavilion on the left. Follow the narrow path with a hedge on the left and wooden buildings on the right, to a stile. Climb this and continue to follow the next yellow waymarker through the paddocks to a wooden bridge and second stile. Cross these and turn left along the field edge. Continue ahead along the well-marked path going between a gap in the hedge, maintain direction

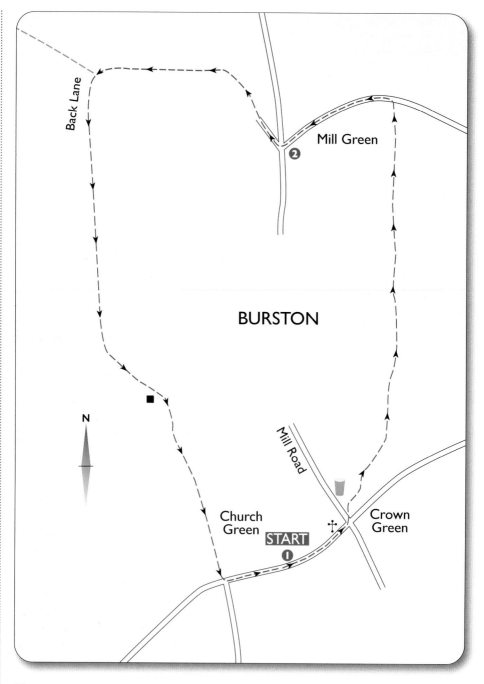

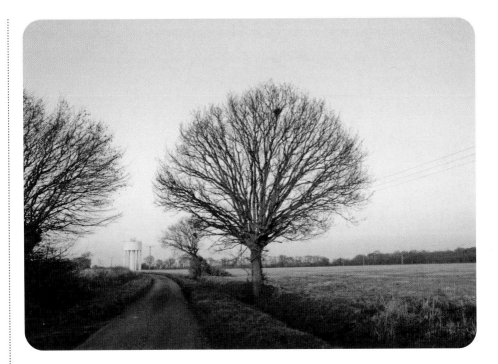

■ *Along the way* ■

across the second field to reach the wide gap in the hedge with a house beyond it to arrive at a country lane. Turn left along the lane and walk ahead, passing Ivy Cottage and the Old Granary to reach the junction at **Mill Green**. The plaque on the corner of this road records that Tom and Kitty Higdon lived here until the death of Tom in 1939.

2 Turn right at the junction, then keep left where the road forks, signposted The Heywood. Continue ahead, then turn left on reaching **Back Lane**. Walk this narrow lane, turn left at the footpath sign, just before the pink-washed house. Walk through the field with crops on either side, continue ahead with trees on the left and stabling on the right to reach a T-junction of paths. Turn right along the track, this can sometimes be very muddy. Continue on the track with a ditch on the left to reach a road. At the time of writing there were three donkeys housed in the stabling on the right. Turn left onto Diss Road, crossing over the road to the pavement. Follow this road going over the bridge with a small stream underneath, walk ahead to return to the start of the walk.

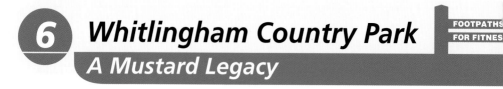

6 Whitlingham Country Park

A Mustard Legacy

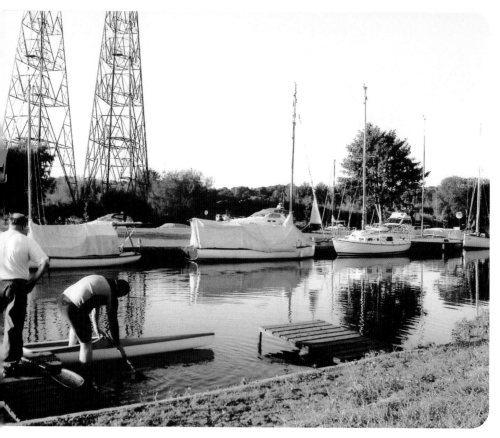

■ *Sailers, canoeists and windsurfers all use the park's amenities* ■

The last of the shorter walks is around the Great and Little Broad, within Whitlingham Country Park. There are several benches and viewpoints to make the most of this walk. Less than 2 miles from the centre of the city of Norwich, there are many activities available here reflecting the growing emphasis on fitness for all. The Outdoor Education Centre offers a variety of wildlife programmes linked to the National Curriculum for use by primary and secondary schools. It also offers courses for all ages in sailing, canoeing and windsurfing.

GRADE: 1
ESTIMATED CALORIE BURN: 225

Terrain: Flat country lanes, one short uphill section, and a riverbank path.
Distance: 2½ miles
Stiles: None
Time: 1¼ hours
Starting point: The visitor centre pay and display car park, Whitlingham Country Park. GR 257078.
How to get there: From the city of Norwich, follow signs for Trowse on the south-east side of the city, then the brown tourist signs for Whitlingham Country Park. Turn left down Whitlingham Lane and follow signs for the Little and Great Broad which are just north of the junction of the A47 and the A146.
OS Map: Explorer 237 Norwich
Refreshments: Whitlingham visitor centre café is highly recommended. It is open all year round at weekends, and daily from April to October. Dogs are welcome and are even given doggie chews!

The Whitlingham Country Park site was once part of the Crown Point Estate, owned by the Colman family of Norwich who are famous for their English mustard. The site has ancient chalk workings and evidence of palaeolithic and neolithic flint knapping. The broads are the result of the flooding of quarries used to extract chalk and gravel for building projects, including the Norwich southern bypass and the development of the Castle Mall shopping centre. Whitlingham Woods which can be seen close by, once provided chalk, transported by wherries from its quarries, for the cement works downstream on the river Yare at Berney Arms and Burgh Castle.

Although the country park is still under development, it is already an important wildlife reserve. It is home to wading birds, terns, many kinds of wildfowl, butterflies and dragonflies. A birdwatching screen overlooks the zoned area for wading birds, with a nesting island for terns.

1 Walk from the car park towards the **Great Broad**. (If using the overflow car park, walk ahead to the car park next to the visitor centre). Turn left at the fingerpost marked 'Wherryman's Way', which is a recently-established path running from Norwich to Great Yarmouth. It is 18-miles long and traces the route used by the trading wherries along the River Yare. Continue ahead

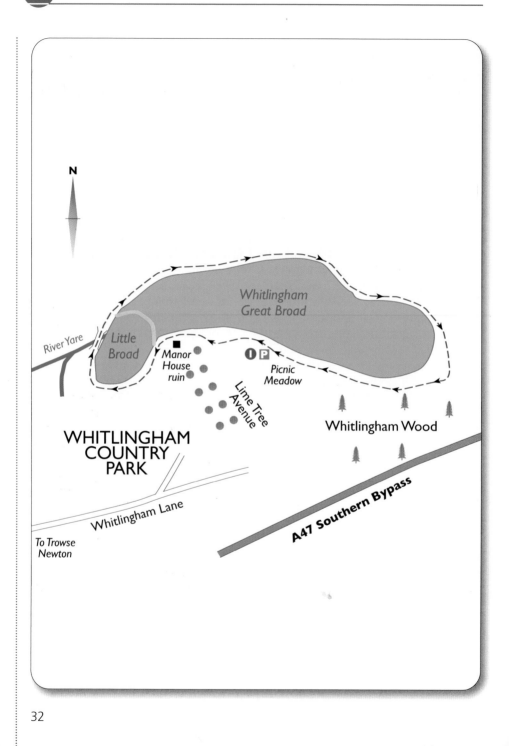

N

Whitlingham
Great Broad

River Yare

Little
Broad

Manor
House
ruin

ℹ️ 🅿️

Picnic
Meadow

Lime Tree Avenue

**WHITLINGHAM
COUNTRY
PARK**

Whitlingham Wood

Whitlingham Lane

To Trowse
Newton

A47 Southern Bypass

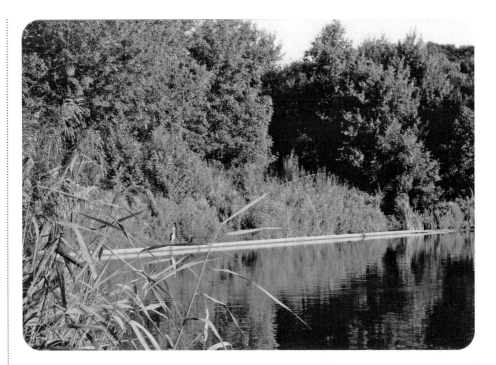

■ *Heron and all manner of wildfowl can be spotted on the water* ■

with the Broad on the right, passing the picturesque ruins of a medieval manor house covered in ivy, then, as the path bends left, go straight ahead through the double wooden gates. This is Little Broad. Maintain direction keeping the Great Broad on the right as the path bends and passes the **Outdoor Education Centre**. Keep on the shingle path to the left of the centre and continue ahead, with the Broad on the right and the **River Yare** now on the left. Follow the path with the conservation area on the right, including a bird screen. This specially-zoned area can be visited by walking a very short distance following the signs, then retracing your steps to the main path. Continue on the path as it bends right to eventually arrive back at the start of the walk. There are countless ducks, swans and geese to be seen along this last part of the walk.

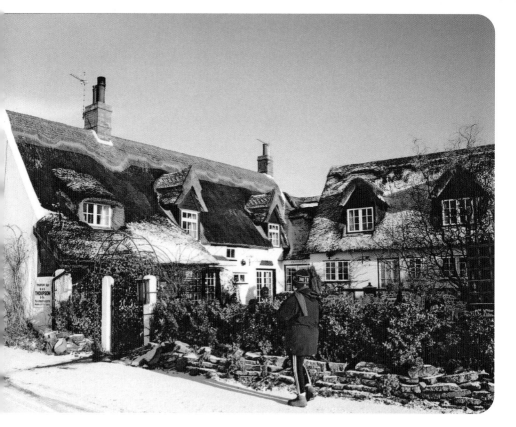

■ *The Staithe 'N' Willow restaurant* ■

Horning is a very picturesque village situated on the banks of the River Bure and makes for an extremely pleasant walk of slightly greater length than those featured thus far. Horning is a very popular village with holidaymakers and sailing enthusiasts and there are a number of private inlets off the river leading to some very attractive properties. This route takes you along the riverside bank then, via a winding lane, to the parish church and the peaceful staithe on the River Bure. In season you can take a Mississippi River Boat ride on the *Southern Comfort* which is moored at the quay near the Swan Inn.

1 Walk from the car park towards the **Swan Inn** and follow the pathway around the front of the inn with the river on the right. Walk along the pathway passing the river green on the left with the small staithe on the right. Continue past the tearooms, turning left to **Lower Street**, then right along it. To view **Hobbs Mill**, turn right at the signpost for the marina. This is an open-framed trestle wind pump which is now a holiday home, alongside it is the very attractive Dutch House, also used for holiday accommodation. Retrace your steps to the road. Continue walking along the road with inlets visible to the right leading down to the river. There used to be a chain link ferry here to Cockshoot Dyke and Broad. Foot passengers can still take the dinghy service to Cockshoot Broad, which has an abundance of wildlife. Continue on past **Ferry Road**, walking out of the village. Just before the school sign look for the metal barriers on the left at the start of a pathway, go around the barriers and follow the path to the road.

2 Cross the road, keeping the village school on the left and walk along the lane signposted 'to the church'. Go through the wooden gates into the churchyard. Walk directly ahead across the grass, following the sign to the narrow enclosed path running behind the east of the church. Follow the path as it slopes downward, there is wooden fence on the right-hand side. Continue down the steps and go through the two gates to the boardwalk and the old staithe. There is a well-placed memorial seat on the staithe for

GRADE: 2
ESTIMATED CALORIE BURN: 170

Terrain: Flat walking along the riverside, country lanes and footpaths, with a short section of wide steps to and from the River Staithe.
Distance: 3 miles
Stiles: None
Time: 1½ hours
Starting point: The pay and display car park by the Swan Inn. GR 340176. Charges vary according to time and season.
How to get there: Horning is situated 3 miles east of Wroxham on the A1062. It is clearly signposted off the A1062.
OS Map: OL 40 The Broads
Refreshments: There are several opportunities for refreshment in Horning. We can recommend the excellent Staithe 'N' Willow restaurant on the river front; there is also the Swan Inn, a good public house near the start of the walk. The Ferry Inn, just off the walk is also open all year.

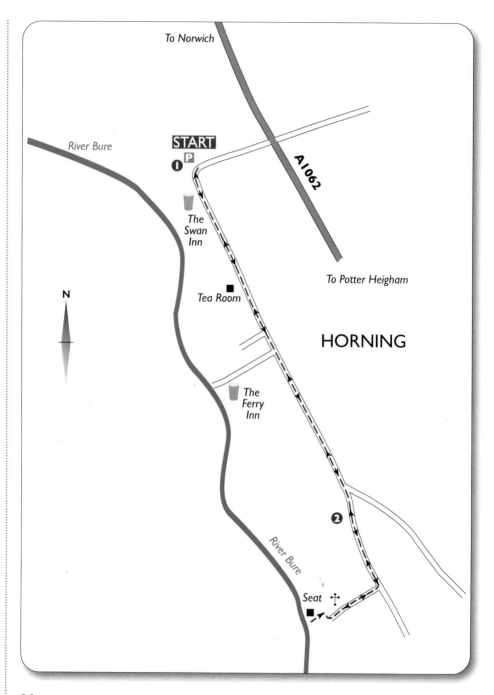

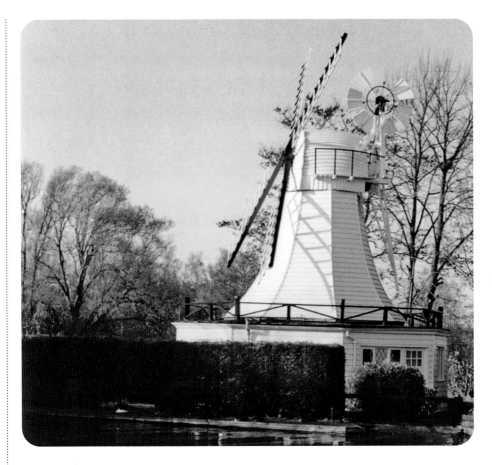

■ *Hobbs Mill at Horning* ■

those who wish to enjoy the beautiful views and the sight of wildfowl in their natural surroundings. When you are ready to leave, return to the church, noticing the lovely rectory as you go. Retrace your steps along the country lane, passing the colourfully-painted school again, and cross the road once more to follow the pathway beside the lane and then the road walked earlier. As you pass, you can visit the **Ferry Inn** by walking down Ferry Road. The inn was rebuilt after suffering a direct hit from a German bomber on 26th April 1941, with the loss of 21 lives. The lone bomber was thought to have seen the lights of a car winding its way to the inn. Retrace your steps if you have visited the inn, otherwise continue ahead along Lower Street to return to the car park. There are many pretty cottages and gardens to admire along the road.

8 *Oxborough*

A National Treasure

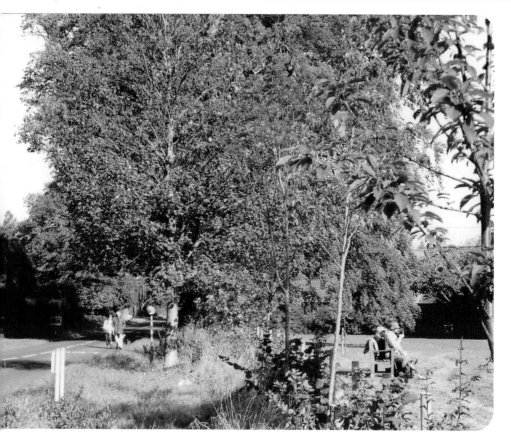

■ *Taking a break on the walk* ■

This simple walk starts from Oxburgh Hall, a National Trust property that is considered to be one of Norfolk's greatest treasures. This beautiful, moated 15th-century house is hidden from view amongst the arable farmland that surrounds it.

The hall has survived centuries of political upheaval. The Bedingfeld family who have owned the property since the 15th century were committed Catholics and loyal Royalists who often found themselves on the 'wrong side'. From the 1570s until 1791, when legal restrictions were at last removed, Catholic services were held in secret. Henry Bedingfeld had a priest hole built to hide the priests. If the washing was left out, this was a signal that a service was taking place.

After the Second World War the estate was sold off. A timber merchant planned to demolish the hall, but Sybil, Lady Bedingfeld, who had married into the family in 1904 managed to buy it back. In 1952 it was given to the National Trust for the nation, however, the Bedingfeld family are still in residence after 500 years. A visit to both the hall and its beautiful gardens is highly recommended.

St John the Evangelist church has been partly ruined since 1948. The original tower with a stone spire was lost to a lightning strike; its replacement lasted 70 years after which the tower and spire again collapsed destroying the nave roof.

1 Walk to the crossroads by the church and then walk along **Eastmoor Road**. After 700 yards, take the footpath on the right, going diagonally across the field on the well-marked path, maintain direction across a second field to reach a sandy track.

2 Turn left along the track. Walk ahead on the track to eventually reach a lane and turn right along the lane at **Caldecote Farm**. There are earthworks of the old St Mary's church in the field. Continue to follow the lane as it bends sharply right towards Gooderstone and Oxborough. Walk ahead to the crossroads, maintaining direction straight ahead, along the country lane.

GRADE: 2
ESTIMATED CALORIE BURN: 310

Terrain: Flat, well-maintained paths and country lanes
Distance: 3¼ miles
Stiles: 3
Time: 1¾ hours
Starting point: Near the entrance to Oxburgh Hall on the grass verge or in the National Trust free car park. GR 744014
How to get there: Oxburgh Hall is on a minor road 6 miles south-west of Swaffham.
OS Map: Explorer 236
Refreshments: Try the excellent National Trust tea rooms at the hall, or the Bedingfeld Arms on the green in Oxborough.

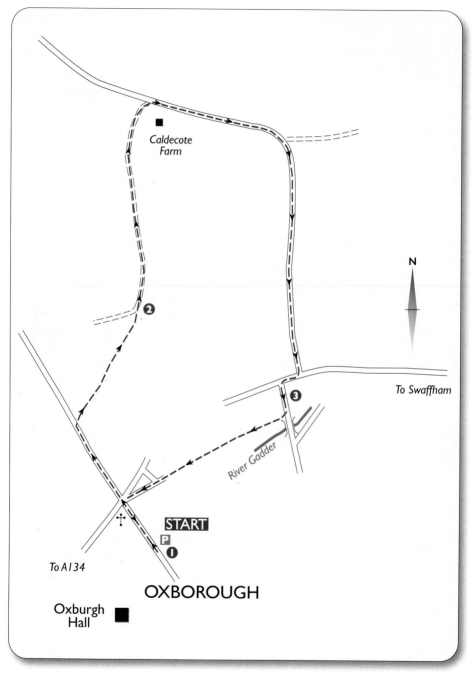

Caldecote
Farm

N

2

To Swaffham

3

River Gadder

START

P

1

To A134

OXBOROUGH

Oxburgh
Hall

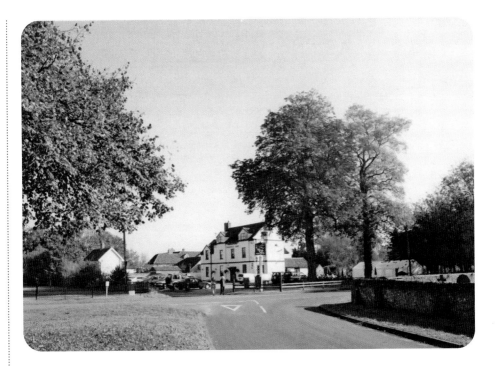

■ *The Bedingfeld Arms on the green at Oxborough* ■

3 Just before the bridge over the River Gadder and next to the Anglian Water Works, look for the footpath sign on the right. If you have time and energy, you could walk a little further over the bridge into the village of **Gooderstone**. The Water Gardens are open every day and are signposted in the village. The rood screen in the church is believed to be one of the best in the country. Retrace your steps over the bridge to continue the walk. Climb the stile and walk straight ahead across the meadow, continue until you reach another stile in the corner of the field. Climb this and continue ahead with a hedge on the left until you reach a third stile, Oxburgh Hall can be seen ahead of you.

Go over the third stile to a path, this leads to a track which emerges at the green, turn left to return to the hall, passing the **Bedingfeld Arms** on the left.

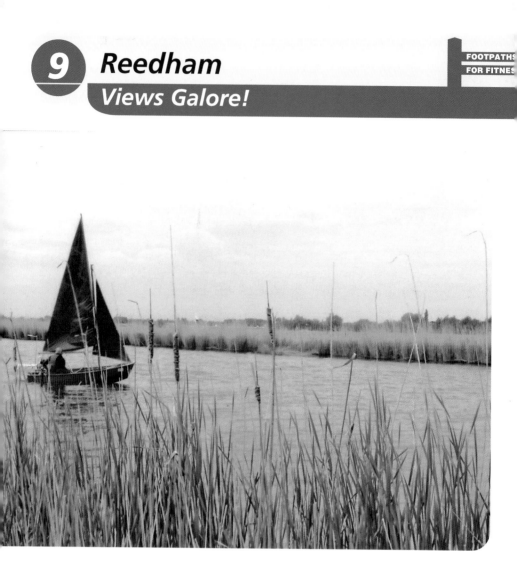

■ *The River Yare* ■

Enjoy a walk around the airy landscape surrounding the fine Broadland village of Reedham. In winter the landscape of river and marshes is quiet, with an ethereal beauty, in summer holidaymakers arrive often by boat giving a liveliness which only adds to its charm. This walk uses the path beside the River Yare, where birds and wildfowl can be seen. It continues to the historic parish church and returns through the village to the start of the walk. There are places to rest and admire the views as you follow the route.

1 From the station car park, cross **Station Road** into **Ferry Road** and follow this for ½ mile to reach the **Ferry Inn**. Across the marshes is the towering Cantley sugar beet factory. Constructed in 1912, it took advantage of the access afforded by both the River Yare and the existing railway. Reedham Ferry operates from next to the Ferry Inn. This last remaining chain ferry used by foot passengers and vehicles to cross the river is a great tourist attraction.

2 Climb the steps from the car park and turn left along the bank, continue walking along the well-defined permissive path passing through two wooden gates. This is a beautiful stretch of the river where it is possible to see the rare marsh harrier as well as the yachts and holiday cruisers. The path also passes a former windmill, now a pretty home with a beautiful garden. Follow the footpath as it bends left, goes down some steps and then turns away from the river to meet a road.

3 Turn right here and continue along **Station Road**, passing several pretty cottages. Keep to the right of the war memorial and continue alongside the river.

The memorial is to the men and one woman of Reedham who perished in the two world wars. It is tragic to note that one name, Hall, appears four times. Three brothers of the family died whilst serving in the First World War. Their sister, Annie, served in France as a nurse. She survived the war but died of influenza and is buried in a British cemetery at Pas de Calais.

GRADE: 2
ESTIMATED CALORIE BURN: 370

Terrain: Flat country lanes, footpaths, one very short uphill path and riverbank walking.
Distance: 3½ miles
Stiles: None
Terrain: Flat country lanes, footpaths, one very short uphill path and riverbank walking.
Time: 1¾ hours
Starting point: Reedham railway station free car park. GR 413022
How to get there: Reedham is 6½ miles off the A47 between Norwich and Great Yarmouth. It is signposted from Acle.
OS Map: Explorer OL 40 The Broads
Refreshments: There are three public houses on the route, together with the Station Café close by the station. The village shop is open daily.

Set in the lawn nearby is a further memorial to the crew of two American bomber aircraft lost at Reedham in 1944 whilst returning to the nearby airfield during the Second World War.

As the road bends left keep straight ahead through the car park of the **Ship** public house, going under the railway bridge, follow the lane a short distance then turn left up a steep but short hill. At the top turn right.

4 Continue along this country lane, which passes several large houses and then bends left. Walk ahead along **Low Common** to reach the railway line leading to Yarmouth. Cross this with care at the single gates and walk along Church Dam to the parish church seen ahead on the right. The church of St John the Baptist is worthy of a visit, the interior contains a section showing the Roman tiles used in its construction. Originally thatched, much of the church was destroyed by fire in 1981, although the 16th-century tomb of the Berney family was rescued. Fund raising by the local population contributed to its rebuilding. Two new stained-glass windows were added in 1999.

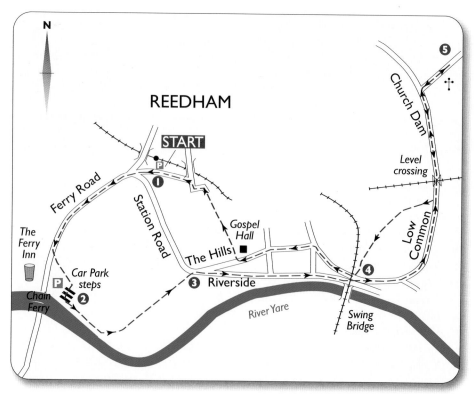

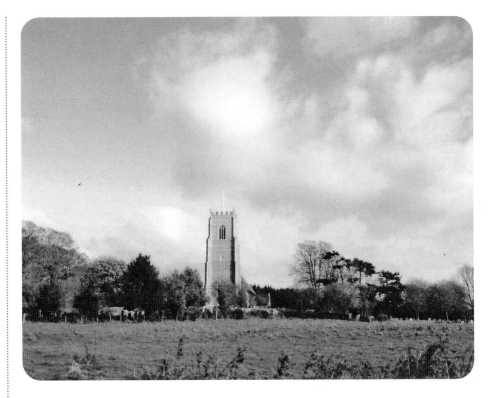

■ *Reedham church* ■

5 After visiting the church, retrace your steps to the railway and cross this again, with care. Once over the line, turn right along a footpath. At its end turn right again and cross the railway bridge. Walk to the junction, passing the village school on the left, cross ahead into **The Hills**. Continue along this road then turn right at the footpath sign and metal barrier, just before the war memorial. At the end of the path turn left into **Witton Green**, then, before the narrow railway bridge, turn left again into **The Havaker**, with the railway line on your right. Walk along **The Havaker** to arrive back at the railway station and the start of the walk.

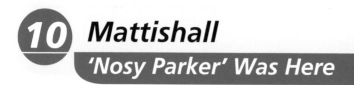

10 Mattishall

'Nosy Parker' Was Here

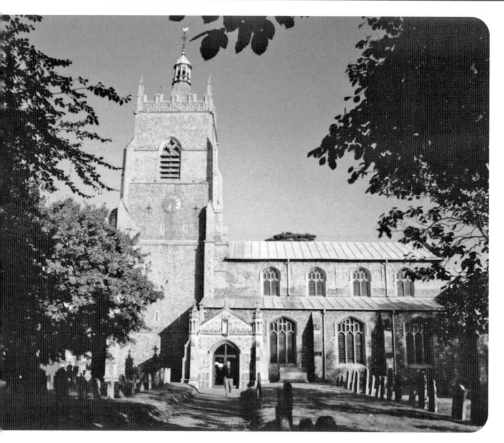

■ *Mattishall church at the start of the walk* ■

This lovely rural walk starts from the magnificent church of All Saints in the pretty village of Mattishall. The route, via peaceful footpaths and lanes, gives ample opportunity to enjoy views of the surrounding countryside.

Mattishall was known for its wool market and many of the quiet lanes here were once sheep droves. The village sign at the beginning of the walk was erected in 1984. Each of the four panels is headed with a different spelling of the village name and various historical characters or events. The front panel depicts Matthew Parker, Archbishop of Canterbury in the 16th century, whose assiduous enquiries of the clergy, it is said, earned him the nickname 'Nosy Parker'. Born in Norwich, he married Margaret Harlestone of Mattishall.

1 From **Church Plain**, walk, with the church on the right, along the 'No Thro Road'. Just before **Talbot House**, turn left along a narrow path; there is a white waymarker on the wall. Turn left again, still following the path, with a fence on the right. The path continues past a school and playing fields and then becomes a covered track with netting on either side. Cross over the concrete bridge at the path end to the field, turn right along the field edge towards a copse, walk through this to the next field and take the path on the right along the field edge, going over a plank bridge. Continue on the path, ignoring another plank bridge and path on the right. Follow the field edge as it turns left, ignore the first path on the right, after a further 20 steps turn right between two hedges to arrive at a country lane, passing **Ebernezer Cottage**.

2 Turn left along the lane, then as the road bends left, continue straight ahead by the footpath sign along the green track, there is a very attractive house on the right. This may be one of the sheep drove tracks. Mattishall had many wool dealers as well as its wool market. Wool was bought in the west of Norfolk to sell through Norwich market. However, some of the dealers flouted the law by selling directly to clothiers. They earned the title of

GRADE: 2
ESTIMATED CALORIE BURN: 310

Terrain: Flat walking along footpaths and country lanes.
Distance: 3½ miles
Stiles: 1
Time: 1¾ hours
Starting point: All Saints parish church. Park at Church Plain near the unusual village sign. GR 054109.
How to get there: Mattishall village is situated on a minor road off the A47, 8 miles west of Norwich and 8 miles east of East Dereham
OS Map: Landranger 133
Refreshments: The Swan Inn public house. There is an excellent village shop on Church Plain, open seven days per week.

'Broggers' and are shown on another of the panels of the village sign. Keep on this long track to reach a stile. Climb this and continue the short distance to the end of the track, passing a house on the left, to arrive at a country lane. Turn left, continue on this long lane to reach a T-junction, turn left again along another lane. Walk ahead until you reach white concrete and iron posts on the left of the lane.

3 Turn right opposite these onto a track between the fields. Maintain direction with first a hedge and then trees to the left. Look for the yellow marker. Turn left here along the field edge, the tower of **All Saints church** can now be seen ahead. Cross the field heading for the archway in the hedge, go through this, crossing the plank bridge and continue across the meadow towards a gate. Maintain direction, then, by a modern house go through the gate with its waymarker. Go through the second gate to the country lane. Turn right then almost immediately left along the green path with a wooden post and rail fence on the left, follow the path round to the right going over the bridge to the field, cross this to the gap in the hedge. Turn right out of

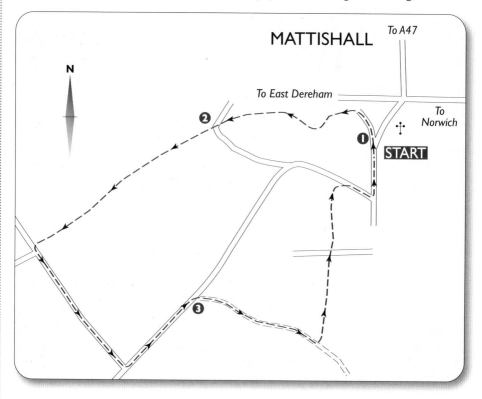

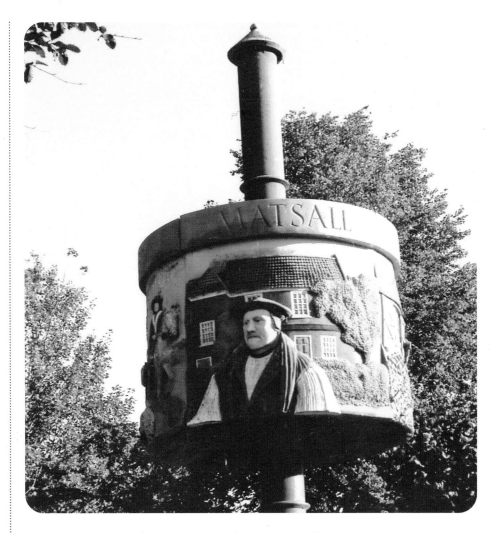

■ *Bishop 'Nosy Parker' on the village sign* ■

the field at the fenced path on the field edge between the houses, to the road. Turn right along the road then immediately left on the narrow path running behind the substation. Turn left on reaching the road. Walk along this road, passing several attractive houses and gardens to return to **Church Plain**. All Saints church has much of historic interest inside, including a fine hammer-beam roof, a 15th-century rood screen and an unusual font. Visiting it makes a lovely end to the walk.

11 Shotesham
A Picture-Postcard Stride

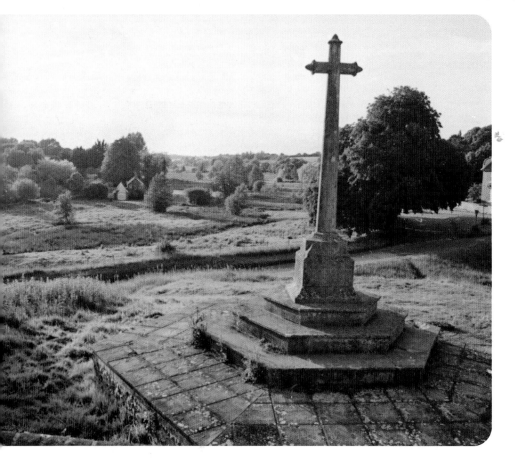

■ *The pretty Shotesham countryside* ■

Shotesham has to be one of the prettiest villages in south Norfolk. Woodland, a ford and wonderful rolling countryside combine to make this walk of increased length a real joy. Those who believe the county of Norfolk to be flat have never been here! The walk takes you from one superb church to another by quiet country lanes and footpaths, then returns passing picturesque cottages, the common and the village duck pond; all of which lure you to complete the walk and burn off the calories.

There used to be four churches in Shotesham but today only three remain: All Saints' church where the walk begins, and St Martin's and St Mary's, both of which are passed later on the walk. William Fellowes, squire of Shotesham in the 18th century, founded the first cottage hospital in England here in the village for use by the eminent surgeon Benjamin Gooch, who is buried at All Saints'. Both of these men were to be influential in the founding of the Norfolk and Norwich Hospital in 1771.

1 From the church, go downhill along **Roger's Lane**, signposted to Saxlingham. Turn left along a track just before some white rails. Follow this path as it goes through the woods and out across a field. Go through a gap in the hedge and over wooden planks. Maintain direction keeping a hedge on the left then, at the end of the field, turn right and follow the path along the left-hand edge of the field until you reach a seat. This is a good place to take a break and enjoy the views of **St Mary's church**. Turn right and continue to the lane, then turn left along it and walk ahead until the next junction, turn right here and continue past the ivy-covered ruins of **St Martin's church**. Continue ahead a short distance, then just before **Old Hall Farm** turn right along the footpath to reach the pretty **church of St Mary** where the churchyard is maintained as a conservation area for wild flowers and fauna. The long grass is cut annually by volunteers from the village.

GRADE: 2
ESTIMATED CALORIE BURN: 420

Terrain: Gently undulating, via paths and lanes.
Distance: 4 miles
Stiles: 3
Time: 2 hours
Starting point: All Saints' church car park at Shotesham. GR 246990
How to get there: Shotesham is located east of the A140 about 6 miles south of Norwich. Follow the signs firstly to Stoke Holy Cross then to Shotesham.
OS Map: Explorer 237 Norwich
Refreshments: The Globe public house, Shotesham. There are tables outside and by the duck pond for use in good weather, a delightful spot for refreshments.

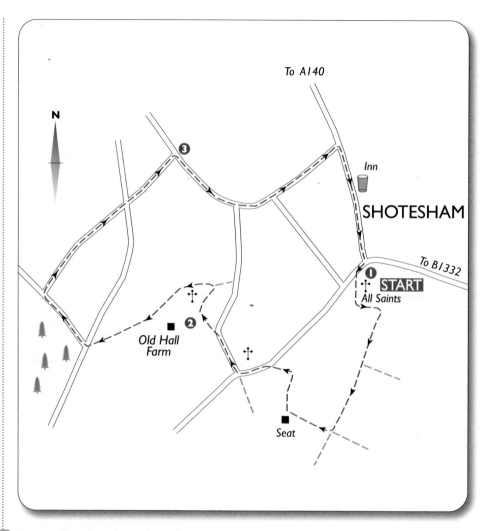

2 Leave the churchyard at the opposite corner and follow the path with a hedge on the left. At the end of the path, climb the stile on the left and cross the field along the clearly-defined path. Climb the next stile into the second field. Climb a further stile into a third field; maintain direction to meet a lane at a junction. The signs for the footpaths here have yellow arrows and are marked 'Norfolk County Council'. Cross the road and continue ahead along the minor road, **Mill Lane**. Turn right at **Knight's Lane** going uphill to a T-junction. Turn left and then immediately right into **Eastells Lane**.

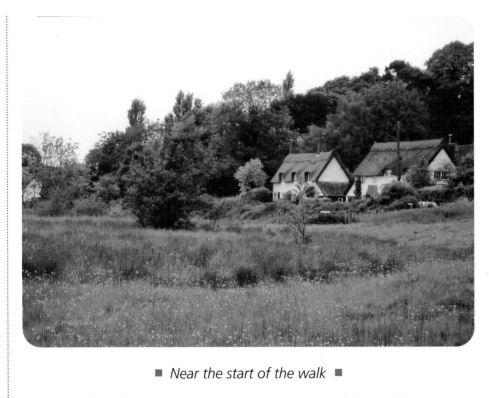

■ *Near the start of the walk* ■

3 Walk ahead to the next T-junction and turn right. Maintain direction to a fork in the road. Take the left-hand fork titled **Hollow Lane** and signposted 'unbridged ford'. Continue ahead passing houses on the left bearing the sign '**St Boltolph's Way**'. St Boltoph was the fourth village church preserved now only in name. Cross over the ford via the footbridge to the road, turn right, passing the Globe public house on the left and the duck pond on the right. Maintain direction to reach All Saints' church and the start of the walk.

12 Fakenham

A Printer's Paradise

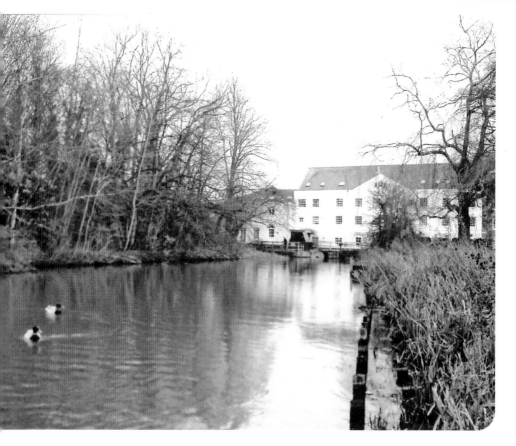

■ *The converted watermill seen on the walk* ■

Starting beside the River Wensum, this walk takes you along its tranquil banks, using part of one of a series of new walks created by Norfolk County Council, then goes into the heart of the town before returning to the start. Fakenham is a very attractive market town. Every Thursday, in addition to the regular market, there is a well-known weekly auction of antiques and furniture.

The town has been a leading centre for printing since the 18th century and this is celebrated in the unusual design of its market square. The pavement in the square contains symbols from the town sign, as well as large metal print plates set into the pavement. The streetlights are representative of pens whilst the seats are designed to echo flowing paper from a printing press.

The Riverside Walk was opened in 2007 and is fully accessible for people of all ages. One of three new paths, it affords the opportunity for everyone to enjoy the countryside whilst also providing health benefits for its users. The river once provided power for three mills, those of Hempton, Fakenham and Sculthorpe, this meant that they all had to work in conjunction as the water headed downstream.

1 Walk over the bridge from the car park and turn left onto the footpath keeping the river on the left, continue on the path until reaching a road. This is a lovely start to the walk, with views of the tower of St Peter and St Paul's church. The tower, at 115 ft, dominates the surrounding area as the church nestles in the very pleasant Georgian heart of Fakenham. At the road turn left and continue for 120 yards. Ahead on the left is a beautifully converted watermill. Cross the road to the **Museum of Gas and Local History**. Continue a short distance then turn right at Fakenham Tyres.

2 There is a sign for the riverside walk here so continue walking ahead keeping the river on the left. Cross the bridge and continue, now with the river on

GRADE: 2
ESTIMATED CALORIE BURN: 400

Terrain: Riverbanks, which can be muddy after rain, and country roads.
Distance: 4 miles
Stiles: None
Time: 2 hours
Starting point: Gogg's Mill Road where there is free car parking over the bridge. GR 913297
How to get there: Follow the A1065 from Fakenham to Swaffham. After the second roundabout take the first left signposted Fakenham Garden Centre and left again to Gogg's Mill Road.
OS Map: Landranger 132
Refreshments: There are various opportunities within the town, including Wensum Lodge Hotel passed on the walk and ideally situated for refreshment whatever the season.

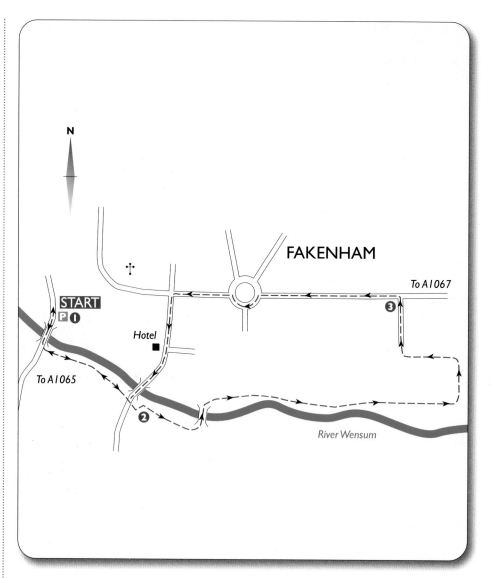

the right. After prolonged rainfall the path can be muddy in places and care should be taken. Eventually walk under a railway bridge. Walk ahead on the track and go over a bridge, there are pine trees on the right as the track leaves the river. At the end of the footpath, pass round the metal gate and turn left. Walk ahead crossing a minor road, into **Barber's Lane** opposite, follow this as it bends right to join **Norwich Road**.

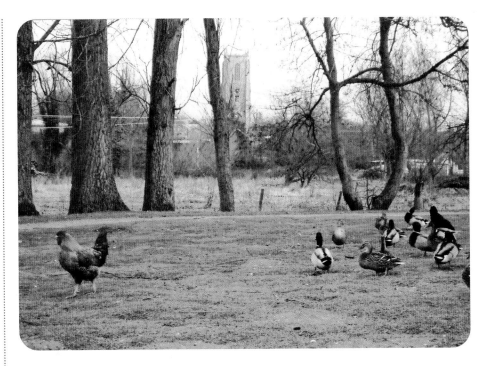

■ *The tower of St Peter and St Paul's church seen through the trees* ■

3 Turn left here and continue straight ahead into the town. Maintain direction going over a mini roundabout, then take the first left into **Bridge Street**. The market square and church are on the right. Continue along Bridge Street then turn right at the mini roundabout. Pass Wensum Lodge Hotel and the converted watermill seen earlier, which is now on the right. Walk ahead and after 150 yards turn right onto the riverside path. Retrace your steps, now with the river on your right, to the start of walk.

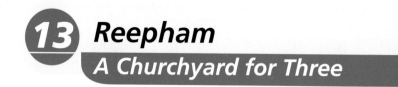

A Churchyard for Three

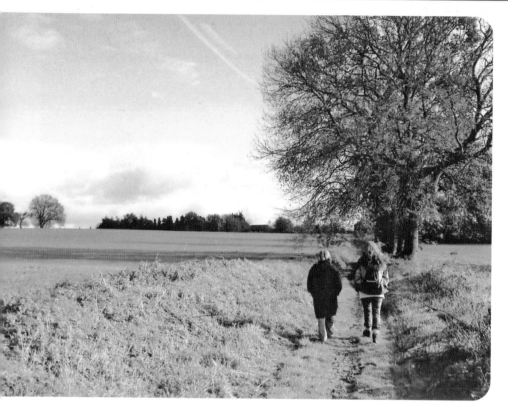

■ *On the outskirts of Reepham* ■

Reepham is a delightful, small market town with an impressive Georgian square and a churchyard, which once housed three churches, two of which remain. The route takes you on a wonderfully rural walk around the perimeter of the town, to its historic centre and narrow alleyways before returning to the start.

The market place is where the three manors of Reepham, Whitwell and Hackford converged. The respective parish churches found themselves necessarily sharing space. All Saints of Hackford is now in ruins, however, the churches of St Mary's, Reepham and St Michael's, Whitwell remain side by side beyond the market place. St Mary's church contains the superb 14th-century tomb of Roger De Kerdeston who died in 1337. The railway arrived in Reepham in 1882, although it failed to bring more growth. The railway closed in 1952 and the former trackbed is now part of Marriott's Way, a long-distance path running from Norwich to Aylsham. It is named after William Marriott, a former chief engineer of the Midland and Great Northern Joint Railway. The old station is now home to a very good tearoom, as well as gift and craft shops.

1 Turn right out of the car park into **Station Road**, then turn left along **Kerdiston Road**, with the Methodist chapel to the right at the corner, continue along this road, passing Smuggler's Lane on the left. Almost 100 yards before the railway-bridge turn left along a track signposted '**Marriott's Way**, Thelmelthorpe Link'. The track has woodland then fields and hedges on either side. Walk ahead on the track to arrive at a road, turn right and then after some 200 yards cross the road and turn left along Broomhill Lane, opposite Wink Cottage. Continue along the lane.

2 Turn right at the edge of the school playing field (before the school is reached) as the path goes uphill. Continue on this path to reach the road. Turn left along it, then right at the top of the hill, walking along a hedged track that bends left at the start and leads to a road. Cross over and continue straight ahead on the lane signposted 'Little Witchingham', passing **Eades Mill** on the left. Eades Mill has an idyllic location, with the River Aisne flowing beneath it. Maintain direction going uphill to reach a road junction.

GRADE: 2
ESTIMATED CALORIE BURN: 430

Terrain: Flat country lanes and footpaths on the old railway line.
Distance: 4½ miles
Stiles: 2
Time: 2 hours
Starting point: Station Road public car park (free). GR 777893.
How to get there: Reepham is on the B1145, 9 miles north-west of Norwich.
OS Map: Landranger 133.
Refreshments: There are several opportunities for refreshment on the walk, including the café at the Old Station, and the Old Brewery House in the market square, both of which we can recommend.

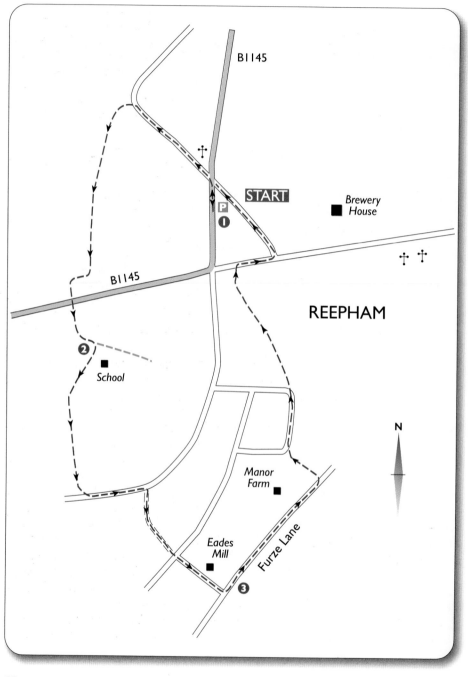

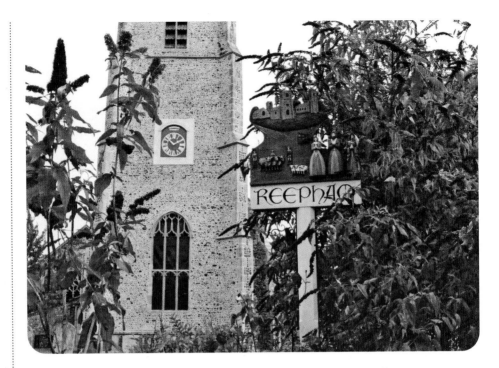

■ *The intriguing village sign in the churchyard at Reepham* ■

3 Turn left, signposted 'Cawston and Booton', this is **Furze Lane**. On a clear day there are superb views of the surrounding countryside and the striking towers of Booton church can easily be seen. If time allows after completing the walk, try to visit this extraordinary Gothic style church, designed by a rector of Booton church. Continue along this road, with the Manor Farmhouse on the left, then turn left at a fingerpost, passing through an iron gate. Continue ahead to cross over a wooden bridge with a stile, climb a further stile at the end of the meadow to arrive at a lane. Turn right and maintain direction passing some pretty cottages on the way. As the lane bends to the left keep straight ahead to a footpath known as Bar Lane. At its end turn left into **Back Street**. Back Street contains many attractive houses, some dating back to the 17th century, including the Greyhound, a former public house. It is worth exploring this street in more detail, then retrace your steps. Turn right into **Pudding Pie Alley** leading to the market place. From here, turn right to visit the two churches. Walk down the narrow lane in the market square between the butcher's shop and the pharmacy to return to the start of the walk.

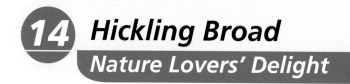

14 Hickling Broad
Nature Lovers' Delight

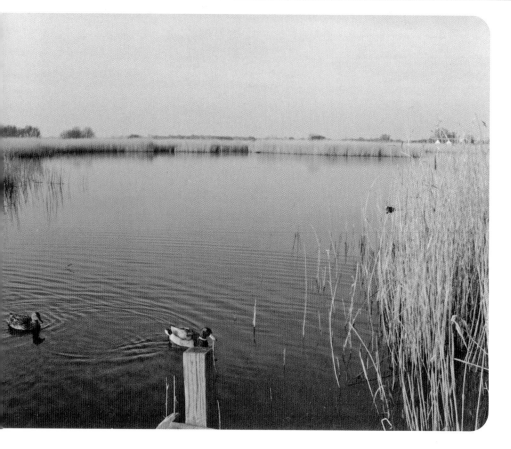

■ *The wonderful reedbeds on Hickling Broad* ■

This wonderful country walk of moderate length passes alongside **Hickling Broad**, the largest of the Norfolk Broads, now owned and managed by the Norfolk Wildlife Trust. Enjoy the peace and tranquillity offered by this walk, with its views of open water, reed-beds and marshland. In season, see the rare swallowtail butterfly, as well as the majestic heron at almost any time of the year. Bring your binoculars if you have some.

The Norfolk Broads are the result of medieval peat digging for fuel. These workings filled with water as the sea rose; the true origins of these wetlands were not discovered until the 1960s. It was not until 1978 that a special organisation, the Broads Authority, was set up to manage them. The dragonfly sign is the emblem of the Broads Authority featuring the rare Norfolk hawker dragonfly, which can be found at Hickling Broad. The Hawker needs unspoiled grazing marsh, dykes, clean water and an abundance of aquatic plants to survive. It can also be found at the nearby nature reserve at Ludham. If you are walking in June or July, look out for the swallowtail butterfly, a protected species since 1981 it is now restricted solely to the Norfolk Broads. On a warm summer's day, you are very likely to see one. It has distinctive yellow and black colouring and extended hind wings, rather like the shape of a swallow's tail. The adult butterflies feed on the likes of ragged robin or thistles, whilst the caterpillars prefer the leaves of the milk parsley which has become increasingly rare in Britain.

St Nicholas church, which is thatched, has a 12th-century round tower, with a 14th-century octagonal top. Inside, it has an interesting rood screen and a tomb chest covered in 17th-century graffiti, including the popular game of nine men's morris. Regretfully the church is currently kept locked due to vandalism.

GRADE: 2
ESTIMATED CALORIE BURN: 400

Terrain: Flat walking along the footpaths and a narrow country lane.
Distance: 4 miles
Stile: None
Time: 2 hours
Starting point: St Nicholas church, Potter Heigham. There is limited parking alongside the church grounds. GR 419199.
How to get there: Potter Heigham is 4 miles south-east of Stalham on the A149. The old village and parish church are on the minor road north of the junction with the A1062. Follow the road to its end and turn right to follow Church Road to St Nicholas church.
OS Map: Explorer OL 40 The Broads
Refreshments: There are no opportunities for refreshments on the walk but there is a well-placed bench by the church for snacks or picnics. Remember to take water with you, especially on a warm day. The holiday area by the medieval bridge, 1 mile away, provides opportunities for refreshments after completing the walk. To reach it, return to the A419 from the direction of the church, turn left and then turn right at the road signs for Potter Heigham.

1 From the front of the church, turn right following **Church Lane** northwards, with the church on the right. Where this narrow lane bends to the left, turn sharply right at the fingerpost and continue along the track. Turn left after 50 yards at the County Council waymarker onto a green lane. Walking toward the woodland, follow the path until you reach the sign and information board on the left for the National Nature Reserve. Turn left into the reserve going through carr woodland and cross over the wooden bridge with the dragonfly sign. Walk up six steps and turn right along **Weavers' Way**. Carr is an area of natural woodland created from unmanaged fen, dominated by willow and alder trees. Follow this well-trodden path with the open water and reed beds on the left and woods on the right. There are

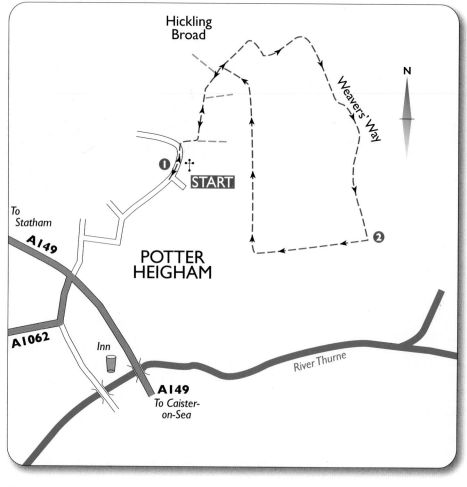

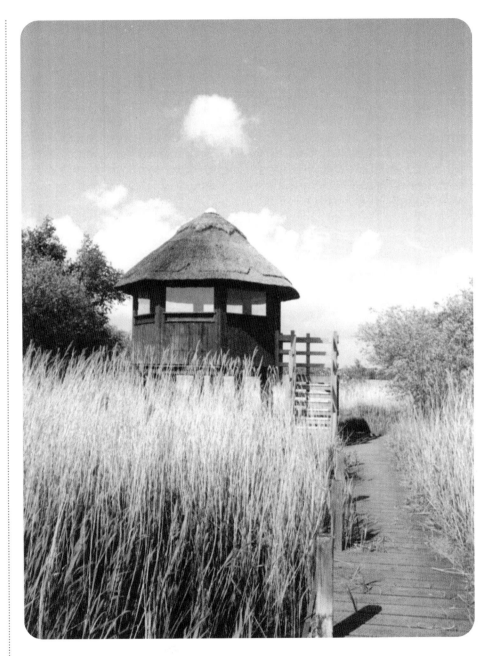

One of the many bird hides in the nature reserve

boarded jetties where you can enjoy the views and appreciate the peaceful surroundings, as well as a hide for birdwatching. Continue on this path for more than a mile to eventually arrive at a gate. Go through this and stay on the Weavers' Way until reaching a wooden footbridge on the right.

2 Cross over the bridge turning right onto a farm track. There are excellent views here of the surrounding marshland and you can often see a heron standing tall and motionless in or near the water. These birds are a magnificent sight in flight with their wings beating very slowly. Stay on the track as it bends left and continues straight ahead. Keep on the track as it bends sharp right, ignoring the green bridleway ahead. Follow the track towards **Oak Tree Farm,** pass this modern red-brick building but do not turn left onto the tarmac lane; instead maintain direction along the track as it narrows and becomes a green lane. Walk ahead and cross the footbridge, continue on the path with a wooden fence on the right. At the end of the fence, continue ahead following the path which eventually returns to the entrance to the nature reserve; ignore this and follow the track taken at the beginning of the walk to return to **St Nicholas church** which can be seen ahead.

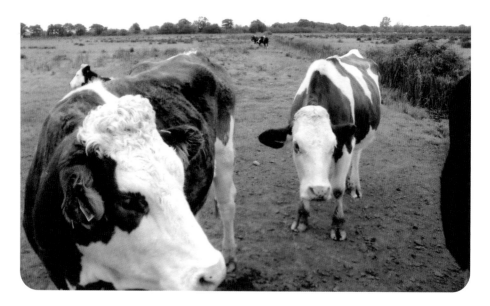

■ *Along the way* ■

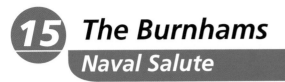

15 The Burnhams
Naval Salute

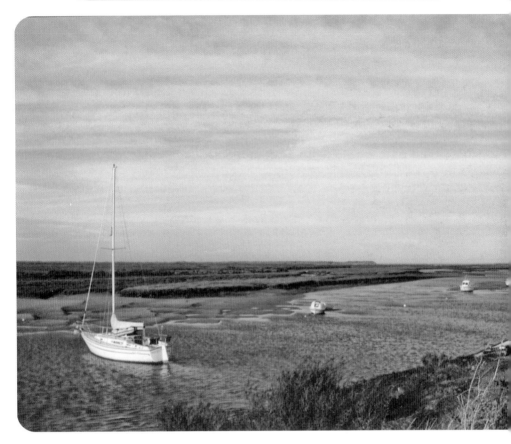

■ *Burnham Overy Staithe* ■

This gorgeous 4-mile walk starts at Burnham Thorpe, the childhood home of Admiral Lord Nelson. It continues on to the beautiful north Norfolk coast path, through a nationally-renowned nature reserve to the picturesque village of Burnham Overy Staithe, and returns by way of Burnham Overy Town. At any time of the year, even in inclement weather, this walk will uplift the spirit as well as helping towards physical fitness.

Horatio Nelson was born in Burnham Thorpe, where his father was rector for almost half a century. The church, widely known as Nelson's church, has much of interest displayed inside about his life; look for the White Ensign and its story. The church of St Clement in Burnham Overy Town is of Norman origin, although the tower includes carr stone indicating an earlier date, and the interior has much of interest. Horatio Nelson would have been familiar with this church as he walked from his home to the staithe to watch the ships.

1 From the church turn right, then after 20 yards turn left through the kissing gate. Continue ahead and climb the stile; then follow the path diagonally through the meadows going over a wooden bridge to a kissing gate. Go through the gate to the embankment and turn left; after a short distance turn right onto a well-defined but unmarked path, down the bank and into a field. With the hedge on the right continue to follow the path over two fields to reach a country road and the village of **Burnham Overy Town**.

2 Cross the road and turn right along it, then, after the last house on the left, turn left along a track. Continue uphill on the track, the extra exertion here will burn more calories! At the path junction turn right and follow the yellow waymarker diagonally right, aiming for the far corner of the hedgerow. (If the field is ploughed, continue ahead at the bottom of the field with its wide grass edge, turn left and with the hedge on the right walk to the yellow marker at the hedge end.) Maintain direction diagonally to the next marker in the hedge gap (or if necessary follow the field edge again) and then to the third sign in the hedge. Go through the hedge to the field, turn right and

GRADE: 2
ESTIMATED CALORIE BURN: 400

Terrain: Flat, mainly on well-defined footpaths.
Distance: 4 miles
Stiles: 3
Time: 2½ hours
Starting point: Burnham Thorpe church. GR 853417.
How to get there: Burnham Thorpe is signposted off the B1155 Wells to Burnham Overy Town road. The lanes leading to it are very narrow and care must be taken whilst driving.
OS Map: Explorer 251 Norfolk Coast Central
Refreshments: The Hero at Burnham Overy Staithe and the Lord Nelson at Burnham Thorpe, both of which welcome walkers.

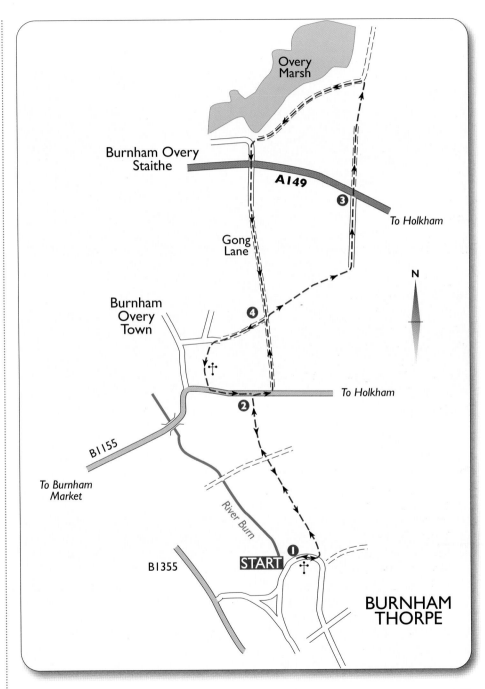

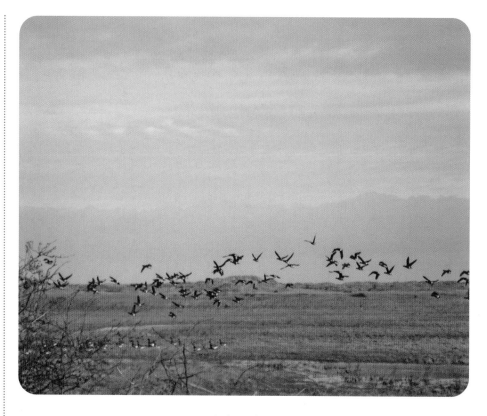

■ *Birds aplenty* ■

walk ahead to reach a narrow country lane. Turn left and continue to the main coast road (the A149).

3 Cross this very busy road with great care and walk straight ahead down the track. Climb the stile to enter the national nature reserve of **Burnham Overy Staithe**. Continue on the track to a stile, after which turn left to reach the staithe. There are wonderful views of Burnham Overy Staithe harbour and windmill on this stretch of the walk, while the creeks and little boats make a picturesque scene. Turn left at the information board of the Burnham Overy Harbour Trust, walk the short distance to the A149. Cross this again with care, then turn left and immediately right to reach **Gong Lane** by the Hero public house. Follow **Gong Lane** uphill for ½ mile. The lane begins as a tarmac path then narrows to become a green lane hedged on either side, until it meets the junction of paths walked earlier.

4 Turn right along the green track and continue until you reach the church at **Burnham Overy Town**, where you turn left at the kissing gate into the churchyard. Leave by the south gate to the road, turn left and walk along the B1155. After 300 yards, turn right at the Burnham Overy parish council sign to the path walked previously. The walk now retraces the route back to Burnham Thorpe church. Continue ahead at the field junction, following the path into the trees, climb the bank and turn left along it. Turn right down the bank at the kissing gate and follow the path through the meadows, crossing the stream and then along the field edge with the hedge on the left. Climb the stile and walk to the kissing gate ahead to return to the start of the walk.

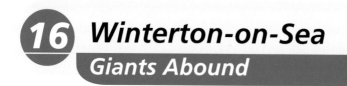

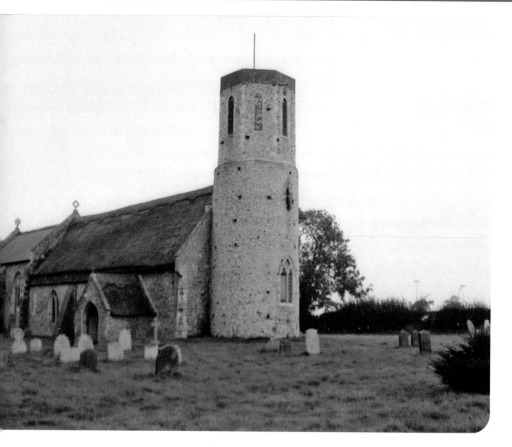

■ *Somerton church* ■

From the gigantic tower of Winterton church, to the resting-place of the Norfolk Giant, this gentle walk passes through a beautiful landscape of traditional wind pumps and a graceful modern wind farm, and returns via a rare coastal acid heath nature reserve.

Holy Trinity and All Saints church has a magnificent 132-ft tower that can be seen from some distance away. Local tradition has it that it stands 'a herring and a half' taller than Cromer church which is said to have the highest tower in Norfolk. The interior contains plaques that record the heroic work of the village lifeboat men in this ancient fishing village. Look for the crucifix carved from a ship's timbers that stands in Fisherman's Corner.

St Mary's church in West Somerton, in its beautiful setting, contains some fabulous 14th-century wall paintings. These were discovered in Victorian times and there are others still hidden by plaster. In the churchyard is the tomb of the Norfolk Giant, Robert Hales, who was born in 1813 in West Somerton and died in 1865. His parents and siblings were all over six feet tall and Robert grew to be 7 ft 8 in. He earned a living with the circus before returning to Norfolk, where he sold penny broadsides containing his life story.

1 Leave the car park and turn left to walk towards the church. At the footpath sign just before the church turn left, walking past allotments, then turn left again at the end of the path. Continue ahead where the track reaches a tarmac lane. The modern wind farm is clearly visible to the left. Follow the lane as it bends left, then at the next left-hand bend take the concrete track straight ahead signed **Low Road**. On the left are the ruins of **St Mary's church**, **East Somerton**, hidden amongst the ivy. It is said that the tree growing inside the ruin originates from a piece of a witch's broomstick. Continue along the track as it bends left and thence to the main road. At the road turn left, walk with care for 200 yards, turning right at **Collis Lane** and almost immediately right again at the footpath sign. Listen carefully to hear the turning blades of the wind farm which boasts ten turbines that have been operating since December 1992. Go through the kissing gate and straight ahead to **St Mary's church** in **West Somerton**.

> **GRADE: 2**
> **ESTIMATED CALORIE BURN: 510**

Terrain: Level tracks, footpaths and country lanes.
Distance: 5 miles
Stiles: None
Time: 2½ hours
Starting point: Winterton Parish Council playing field car park. GR 494195
How to get there: Winterton-on-Sea is situated on the B1159, eight miles north of Great Yarmouth.
OS Map: Explorer OL 40 The Broads
Refreshments: The Fisherman's Return in Winterton-on-Sea.

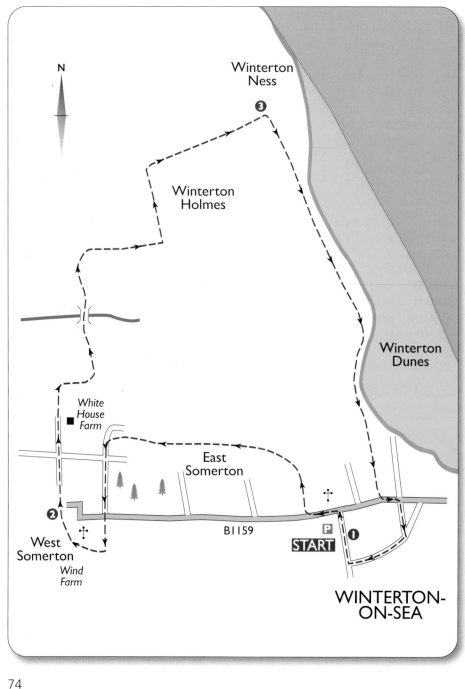

N

Winterton
Ness

❸

Winterton
Holmes

Winterton
Dunes

White
House
Farm

East
Somerton

West
Somerton

❷

Wind
Farm

B1159

START

P

❶

WINTERTON-
ON-SEA

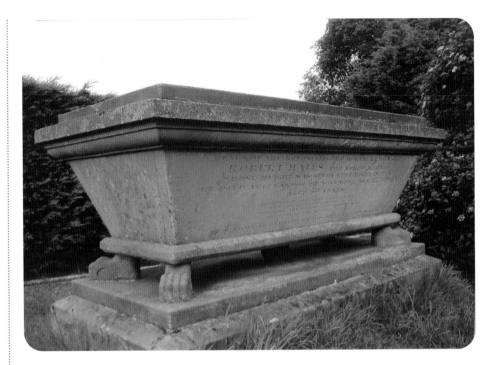

■ *The giant's tomb in Somerton churchyard* ■

2 Leave the churchyard via the lychgate and follow the lane as it bends right to join the B1159. From here there are wonderful views across the landscape. At the main road, by the war memorial, turn right and then left at **The Street**. Maintain direction as the road becomes a concrete path and then a track. Follow the track as it bears right and go through the gate. Continue along the track, then take the left fork with the waymark signs. There are extensive views across the fields and marshland and beyond to the dunes. At the end of the hedge on the left, turn right at the fingerpost next to the tree. Before turning look to the far left for a view of Horsey Mill which is a restored windpump now managed by the National Trust. The path reaches a concrete area with farm buildings. Follow the footpath ahead as signed and then continue along the path until it reaches an iron gate with sand dunes beyond.

3 Walk round the side of the gate and, at the end of the path, turn right at the fingerpost along the sand dunes. The **Winterton Dunes Nature Reserve** is home to rare natterjack toads and is popular with birdwatchers.

There is an information board giving more detail about this important nature reserve. For a view of the sea and a possible sighting of the colony of seals which live nearby, ignore the turn to the right and go straight ahead through the gap in the dunes, then retrace your steps to the fingerpost to continue with the walk. Follow the wide path along the dunes to its end, aiming for the flat roofed white building with blue shutters. Walk ahead into the village, at the Methodist chapel turn left onto **Beach Road** then right into the **Loke**. At its end turn right, then right again into **The Lane**, passing the **Fisherman's Return**, then turn right from the pub or, if just passing it, turn left onto **Black Street** walking back to the church and the start of the walk.

Terrington St John
Wide Skies and Open Spaces

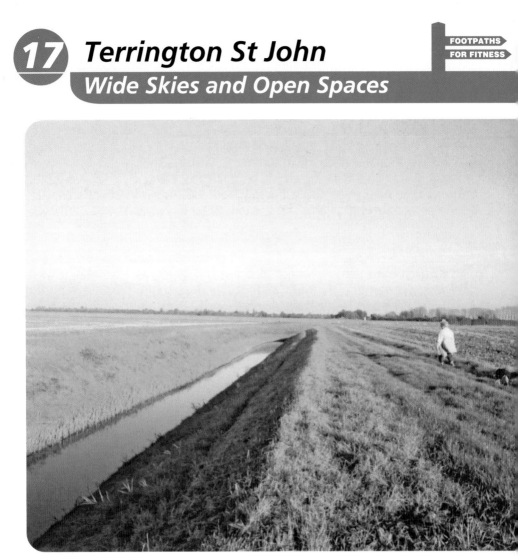

■ *A fine path to get the heart racing* ■

Norfolk is famous for its big skies and this walk in the flat landscape at the edge of the Fenland justifies the fame. The open landscape seems to stretch forever and is dominated by a vast ocean of sky. Once subject to catastrophic flooding, this marshland area is now part of the land reclamation schemes of the 19th century, with deep, wide drainage ditches. An easy walk, the route uses the footpaths alongside the drains and dykes, in a landscape which exudes an atmosphere of quiet calm.

The church of St John the Baptist has a tall tower. Originally the lower stage was open, possibly to avoid flooding, and the tower was separate from the church. The church, which is full of light, has a beautiful west window and a vast 18th-century font. The church forms part of a group known as the Marshland Churches. These include the nearby Terrington St Clement, Walpole St Peter, Walpole St Andrew, West Walton and Walsoken. All of these churches have much to interest visitors. The wealth of the wool industry in this area is reflected in the buildings, ironically they were built during a time when this isolated area was seen as uncivilised and desolate. If time permits, a visit to any of these would be worthwhile.

1 Walk from the church to the road, turn right for 200 yards to the junction with **Church Lane** and turn right along it. Follow the lane for little over ¼ mile passing a farm on the right, until you reach a rough track crossing road with a Second World War pillbox nearby. Turn right along the track which becomes grassy and swings right then left to arrive at a T-junction of paths. Turn right. This is **Fenditch Lane**, which forms the boundary with the neighbouring parish of Terrington St Clement. Continue along the path alongside a wide drain for 200 yards, then turn left going over a concrete

---

GRADE: 2
ESTIMATED CALORIE BURN: 450

Terrain: Flat walking along the footpaths and short sections of country lanes.
Distance: 5 miles
Stiles: None
Time: 2 hours
Starting point: Parish church car park of Terrington St John, north of the A47. GR 540158.
How to get there: Terrington St John is south-west of King's Lynn. Follow the signs from the A47, follow the road signposted Wisbech / Lynn when entering the village. (Terrington St John is divided into two areas.) Follow the main road into the village passing Church Lane on the left. The parish church is further along the road on the left.
OS Map: Explorer 236 King's Lynn, Downham Market and Swaffham
Refreshments: None on the route. We can recommend the Woolpack public house on Main Road on the outskirts of the village south of the A47.

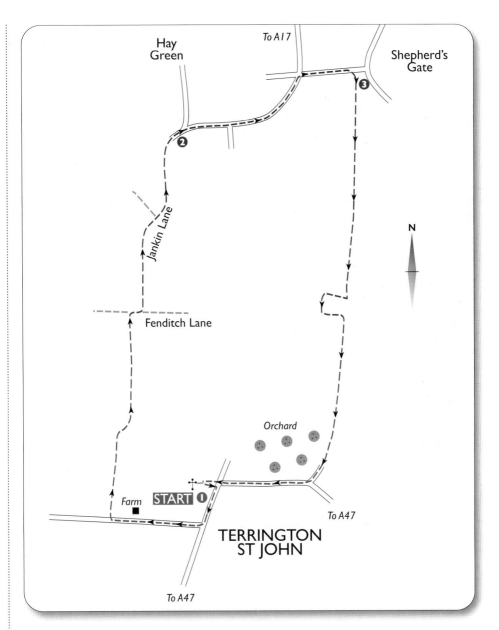

bridge and passing under power lines, aiming for the bungalows which can be seen ahead. The track curves and becomes tarmacked as it approaches the hamlet of Hay Green. Walk ahead to the country lane.

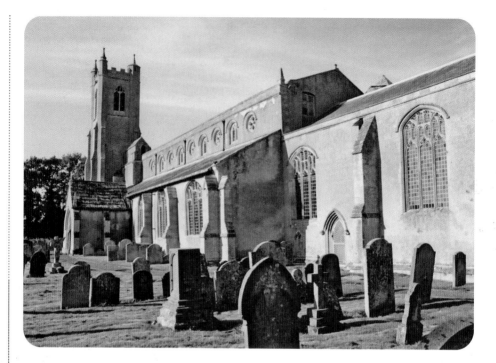

■ *The church of St John the Baptist at Terrington St John* ■

2 Turn right at the give-way sign onto the lane. At the next junction at **Hay Green** turn left onto the main road signposted Terrington St Clement and Lynn. Walk along this busy road with care to a crossroads. Turn right into **Bullock Road** and continue ahead.

3 Just before the next junction at **Shepherd's Gate**, opposite a give-way sign, turn right along the track with a drain on the left. This is **Five Mile Bank**, the parish boundary with Tilney All Saints. The track becomes grassy and eventually reaches a wide drain, the same one crossed earlier on the walk. Turn right for 100 yards, going left over another concrete bridge, then turn left going back to the drain of Five Mile Bank and continue to follow the track walking south with the drain on the left. There are many birds to be seen on this walk, we were fortunate to see several skylarks at this point. The path passes a series of orchards and soft fruit bushes on the right before eventually reaching **Victoria Road**. Turn right along the lane and at the end cross over the main road and turn left to return to the church gates on the right, 100 yards further on.

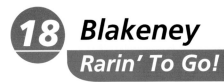

18 Blakeney
Rarin' To Go!

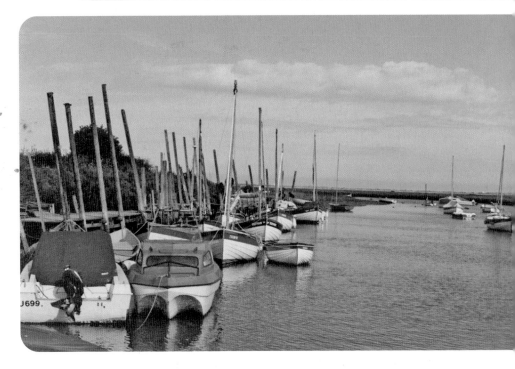

■ *Blakeney harbour* ■

Blakeney, with its natural harbour, dunes, mudflats and colourful waterfront, is a perfect place to start this longer and more challenging walk. There are opportunities to stop and enjoy the stunning scenery, so allow plenty of time to savour its delights. This circular walk takes you via the Norfolk Coast Path from Blakeney to the picturesque village of Cley-next-the-Sea, with its landmark windmill, thence by footpaths and country lanes to the ford at Glandford, an ideal spot for a picnic. A short uphill stretch takes you onto Wiveton Downs, which afford superb views of the coast, before you head back to the start.

The village of Cley was once an important port; in the 14th century it accounted for almost half of the wool exported from the north Norfolk coast. Its restored windmill is a great favourite with artists and it is open to visitors during the summer months.

If you still have some energy and time left after the walk, why not stroll around Blakeney's charming streets. In summer, the gardens, nooks and crannies are filled with self-seeded hollyhocks. The blue plaques on some of the cottage walls relate to the Blakeney Neighbourhood Housing Society. This was formed in 1946 with around 42 homes available to rent at reasonable prices to people born and brought up in the locality.

1 Turn left from the car park onto the **Norfolk Coast Path** which runs along the raised bank opposite the public toilets. Continue along the path for 1 mile, then turn right as the path heads inland toward the village of **Cley-next-the-Sea**. At the end of the path climb the bank, turn right and continue until you reach the A149.

2 Turn left passing Cley Sluice and walk with care along the road for 110 yards. As the main road bears left, turn right (signed to the church) passing the delicatessen on the corner. Continue along the lane past the post office to arrive at **Cley Green**, with the Three Swallows public house on the left. The magnificent parish church of St Margaret is situated on the rising ground to the left, just beyond the pub and is a must to visit. It dominates one end of the village and stands testament to the former wealth and importance of Cley. Take the lane opposite the public house, with the green on the left. At the crossroads continue straight on. Where the road later bends to the left,

---

GRADE: 3
ESTIMATED CALORIE BURN: 720

Terrain: Flat walking on the creek bank and footpaths, one short uphill stretch
Distance: 7 miles
Stiles: None
Time: 3 hours
Starting point: Blakeney Quay where there is a National Trust car park (fee payable). GR 028443.
How to get there: Blakeney is on the A149 between Wells-next-the-Sea and Sheringham.
OS Map: Explorer 251
Refreshments: There are excellent caravan tea stalls at the car park in Blakeney, several teashops in Cley, plus the Three Swallows public house at Cley Green. The Picnic Fayre delicatessen in Cley, passed on the route, is an ideal place to buy picnic food.

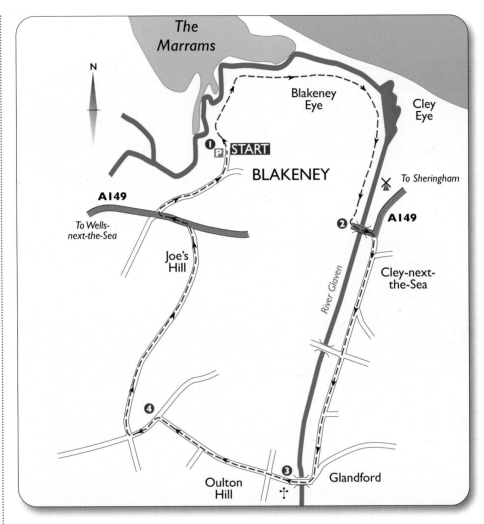

take the right turn signposted 'Unsuitable for motorists'. Once over the ford you are in **Glandford**, an estate village belonging to the nearby Bayfield Hall.

3 Walk ahead passing the pretty parish church and the unusual museum which was built in 1915 by Sir Alfred Jodrell to house his collection of shells, fossils and semi-precious stones. At the junction, cross over the main road to walk uphill on a lane signed 'Langham'. This area is part of the **Wiveton Downs**. In earlier centuries Wiveton rivalled both Cley and Blakeney in its sea trading and fishing, but silting up after land reclamation led to its demise.

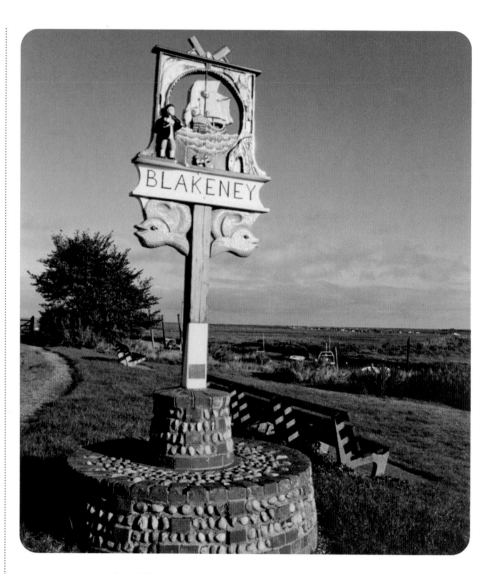

■ *The village sign, with some welcome benches* ■

4 On reaching the T-junction at the top of the hill, turn left and then right at the next junction, signed to Blakeney. Continue along this lane for 1 mile to arrive back at the main road in **Blakeney**. Turn left and then right at the main crossroads. Carry on past the pretty cottages to arrive back at the quay and the car park.

19 *Weeting Castle and Grime's Graves*

Shifting Up A Gear!

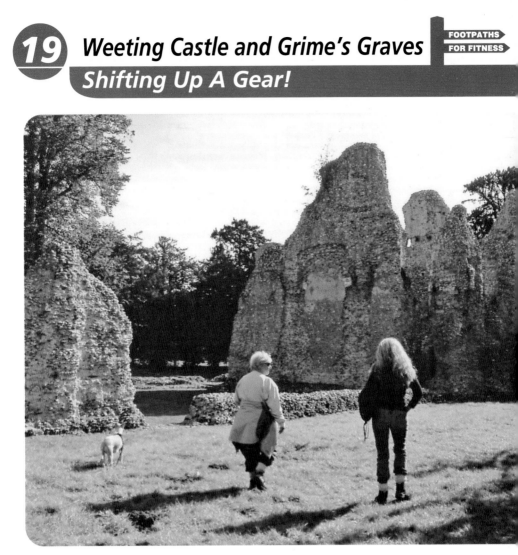

■ *Weeting Castle* ■

One of the longer walks, this provides differing scenery as it takes you through attractive woodland, then across heathland to the Neolithic site of Grime's Graves and returns via forest trails. The walk includes the picturesque ruins of Weeting Castle and the delightfully restored church of St Mary. The terrain is flat which is an advantage for this lengthier walk, we recommend you take water with you and allow yourself time to enjoy your increasing fitness.

Grime's Graves is at the heart of this beautiful scenery and the atmosphere is pleasantly eerie. Despite its name this is not a burial ground, it is derived from the Anglo-Saxon Grims quarries, or Devil's Hole. At 5,000 years old, these Neolithic flint mines are one of the earliest industrial sites in Great Britain. The origin of the mysterious hollows remained undiscovered until they were excavated in 1870. English Heritage now manages the site. There is an admission charge to the exhibition at the centre and to the mineshaft.

Weeting Castle was constructed in the late 12th century, but unlike the motte and bailey castle seen at Castle Acre (*Walk 1*) this was not constructed with serious defence in mind. Whilst built in the style of a castle, it was intended as a manor house complete with a great hall and surrounded by a moat; a surprising amount of the castle remains today and the ruins are still impressive. The castle, thought to contain flint from the nearby Grime's Graves, is now under the protection of English Heritage. It is open all year and entry is free of charge.

St Mary's church in Weeting has been beautifully restored, it stands on a slight rise and has bright red gates erected in memory of the fallen of the Second World War. Its 19th-century restoration was thanks to John Julius Angerstein, the owner of Weeting Hall. An eminent banker for Lloyds, he was a great patron of the arts and upon his death the House of Commons voted to purchase 38 of his pictures at the cost of £57,000. These were to form the foundations of the National Gallery.

GRADE: 3
ESTIMATED CALORIE BURN: 700

Terrain: Flat walking along the footpaths, forest trails and country lane.
Distance: 7½ miles
Stiles: 2
Time: 3 hours
Starting point: Weeting parish church. There is parking at the lay-by at Weeting Castle next to the church. GR 777893.
How to get there: Weeting village is off the A1065, 2 miles north of Brandon, follow the English Heritage signs for Weeting Castle.
OS Map: Explorer 229 Thetford Forest in The Brecks
Refreshments: The visitor centre at Grime's Graves sells soft drinks and hot drinks, together with sweets, biscuits and crisps. There are picnic tables and we recommend that you take a packed lunch.

1 Walk along the lane away from the castle and pass the round church tower, following the track to **Home Farm**. Continue on the broad farm track as it bends, then at the corrugated iron structure on the right and near a Weeting Village Walk waymarker, turn right along the straight track, passing the house on the right. Continue past an open space where the track then forks, follow the Walk sign again and turn right and then left walking on the straight track, with trees on the left, to arrive after almost a mile at the A1065.

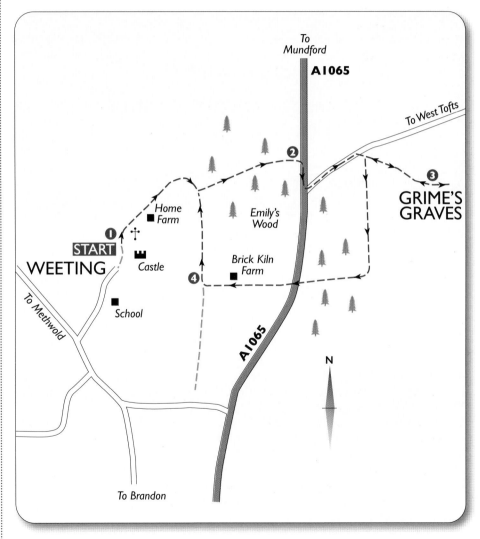

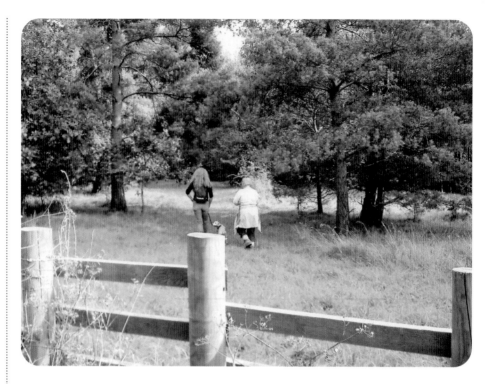

■ *Stepping out on the route* ■

2 Turn right along the road, there is a very wide grass verge for walking. Cross the A1065 when opposite the turning for West Tofts and Grime's Graves. Please take great care when crossing, as the traffic moves very quickly on this straight road. Continue along the lane towards **Grime's Graves**, eventually passing some white metal gates on the right; then look out for a wooden stile and footpath on the right. Climb the stile and walk through the trees to the clearly defined grass path ahead, follow this over the open heathland to the pine trees ahead. Stay on the path as this area forms part of the Ministry of Defence armed forces training ground. The solitary visitor centre building and car park of Grime's Graves, appear ahead as you approach the copse. Go right of the trees and through the kissing gate, turn left and walk to the corner of the fencing, then turn right keeping the fence on the left and walk 100 yards to a stile on the left. Climb the stile and walk towards the visitor centre. We recommend you take a break at this roughly halfway point on the walk to soak up the views and atmosphere and if you have one, enjoy a packed lunch.

3 Leave the centre and retrace your steps all the way back across the heath, climb both stiles again to reach the road once more. Turn left and return to the white metal gates passed earlier, then turn left on to the forest trail at the black and yellow pole, at right angles to the road. Keep on this track, ignoring initial crossing tracks until you reach a crossing track with open ground on the right and a beech tree marked 15½ on the right with a solitary pine to the left. Bear left of the beech tree and walk ahead for 30 yards, then take the right-hand fork (ignore the track to the left). This grassy track has pine trees on the left with deciduous trees on the right and can be very wet. Continue on this path until it emerges on to a sandy lane crossing ahead. There is an oak tree on the right marked '15' about five feet above ground level, turn right along the track and continue for 1 mile to arrive at another black and yellow pole, a track sign (number 24) and the A1065 once more. Cross the road, again with care, and walk straight ahead along the track into the wood, leading to **Brick Kiln Farm**. The path continues beyond some majestic beech trees at the farm. Maintain direction across the field to the hedge ahead then turn right, keeping the hedge on the left.

4 Continue along the track, with a field on the right, going between trees and maintaining direction to regain the outward path. Turn left back along the straight track taken at the start of the walk to return to **Home Farm** and **St Mary's church**.

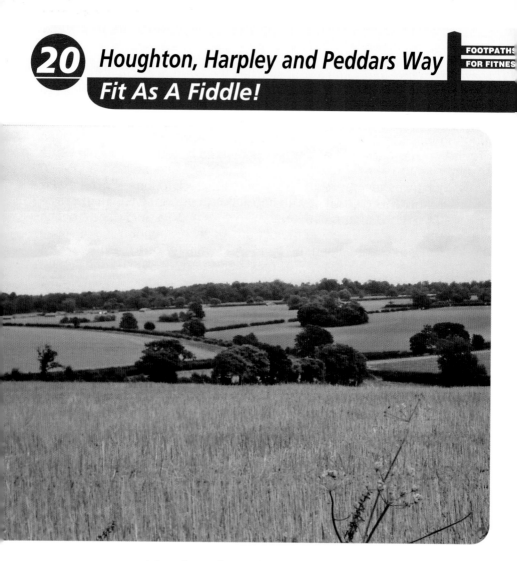

■ *View from the Peddars Way at Harpley* ■

This, the final walk in the book, uses part of a national long-distance path and gives glorious views of the open countryside. It goes through peaceful woodlands and a pretty village, with the added bonus of a view of one of the greatest country houses in the county.

Houghton Hall was built in the early 18th century for Britain's first Prime Minister, Sir Robert Walpole, and was designed in the Palladian style. Walpole created the position of Prime Minister, a post which he occupied for 22 consecutive years. Twice yearly he gave parties which became famous as his Norfolk Congresses. Colleagues in the Government and local gentry assembled in large numbers to eat, drink, hunt and generally indulge themselves. It was said they lived 'up to the chin in beef, venison, geese, turkeys, etc and generally over the chin in claret, strong beer and punch'. He later accepted the property of 10 Downing Street from King George II on the understanding that it would always be the official residence of the Prime Minister.

The Hall, now the home of the Marquis of Cholmondeley, is open to visitors from Easter Sunday to the end of September. If you do not have time to visit the Hall before or after this walk, do come back another day. There is a wonderful walled garden covering five acres, mainly laid out within the last ten years. On our visit in September, visitors were allowed to pick the sweet peas, a lovely touch. Telephone 01485 528569 for more details.

1 Turn right from the parking area walking along the road with the woods on the left. Look for the fingerpost amongst the trees opposite an information board about the **tumulus** you can see here. Many of these burial grounds have been lost through levelling and deep ploughing during the expansion of arable farming from the 1940s to the 1960s. Today, farmers are increasingly encouraged to conserve these ancient sites. Turn left straight

GRADE: 3
ESTIMATED CALORIE BURN: 775

Terrain: Walking mostly on tracks and footpaths, short sections of country lane walking with one main road to cross. The return along Peddars Way is mainly uphill.
Distance: 8½ miles
Stiles: None
Time: 4½ hours
Starting point: Parking is on the grass verge at the crossing point of the Peddars Way long-distance path on the road from Anmer to Harpley. GR 758285.
How to get there: 10 miles north-east of King's Lynn, travel 2 miles north of the A148 on a minor road from Anmer to Harpley.
OS Map: Explore 250 Norfolk Coast West
Refreshments: The Rose public house in Harpley. Take a snack or picnic with you on this walk, there are plenty of stopping points. Water is essential on this length of walk.

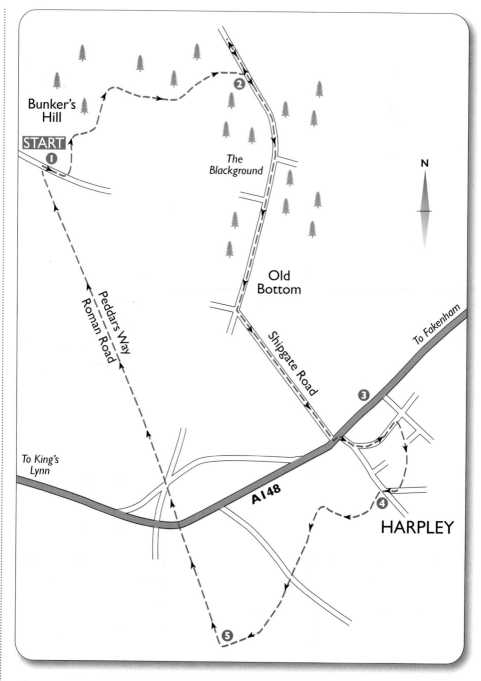

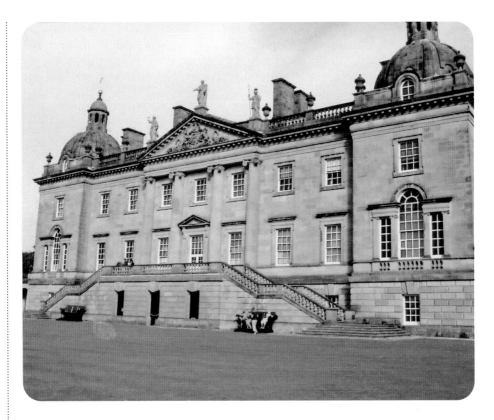

■ *Houghton Hall* ■

into the wood following the well-defined path with yellow waymarkers. Emerge from the wood to a clearing with a footpath sign, you can see a cottage across the field. Turn left and walk around the field edge, ignoring a path into the trees, and follow the grass path heading for the cottage. Pass in front of the cottage and walk along the green lane, which becomes a track, passing a pig farm on the right, and heading towards a farm also on the right. These were some of the happiest pigs we have seen on our walks! They had ample room to move around and made lots of what we believe were friendly grunts as they saw us coming. At the end of the track turn left at the yellow waymarker along the farm drive, follow this to arrive at a country lane opposite a white lodge.

Turn left along the lane for 150 yards for a view of **Houghton Hall**; this view, known as West View looks down a long, wide avenue that stretches on both sides of the road.

2 Retrace your steps to the lodge and then continue ahead down the very quiet road. Where the road bends left, signposted 'Houghton ¾ mile', continue straight ahead down a minor lane, ignore the right turn to Anmer and continue ahead. Turn left at the next crossroads, going uphill, to meet the A148 at the end of this long lane.

3 Cross this main road with great care and go along the road signed to Harpley. Turn left just past the 30 mph sign, into **Raven's Lane**, passing **Harpley Hall**. There is a view of the parish church to the right. Just beyond the Coach House on the left, turn right along the footpath. Follow the track until it reaches a very narrow tarmac lane then turn right along it. Turn left at the footpath just before the trees. Continue downhill on the well-trodden path by the edge of the wood. At the end of the path turn right onto a lane and then right again at the next junction. This is the main road through Harpley. Turn left at the footpath sign by the postbox, into **Brickyard Lane**, or if you wish, continue ahead a short distance to the Rose and Crown on the right and then return to Brickyard Lane. This gravel track shortly becomes a very narrow green path which leads to an open field, walk ahead with the hedge on the right, maintain direction at the next field junction. This ancient track becomes a clearly defined path. Traffic can be seen in the distance ahead. Turn left at the hedge-end going downhill, still on a green track. There is no footpath sign here. On reaching the country lane where the path ends cross over the lane and go through the gateway with a yellow and green waymarker. Continue around the five-bar gate by the trees ahead of you, walk along the track and field edge to the cottage on the left and a farm on the right, turn right along the track. This is **Peddars Way**, the long-distance path covering 46 miles from Knettishall Heath in Suffolk to Holme next the Sea on the north Norfolk coast. It is based on part of the Roman road which ran a similar route.

4 The final section of this walk is entirely on Peddars Way. Continue on the gravel track with hedges on each side to arrive at the A148, by the Dogotel Kennels. Cross the main road very carefully, as it is very busy. Walk ahead along the lane, ignoring the side roads. Maintain direction towards the cottages ahead and continue along Peddars Way. The track climbs uphill for some distance, very good for the fitness levels and calorie burning! The track then passes another tumulus on the right before arriving back at the start.

Calorie Chart

The following chart shows the approximate calories spent per hour by a person weighing 8 stone (112 lbs), 17 stone (238 lbs) and 20 stone (280 lbs)

	8 stone	17 stone	20 stone
Walking, 2 mph	160	240	312
Walking, 3 mph	210	320	416
Walking, 4½ mph	295	440	572

Note that these figures are based on moderate, not vigorous, activity.